T0065322

"A solid contribution to the lives of those who read this phenomenal book and the health industry."

— **Lisa Nichols**, best-selling author and one of the world's most celebrated motivational speakers, is featured in the movie The Secret

"Toni is an excellent guide when it comes to the reversal of autoimmune disorders and chronic illnesses, as well as building new healthy habits that improve quality of life"

—**Lee Holden**, international celebrated QiGong master; well-known television personality who has appeared regularly on PBS

"Toni provides a practical roadmap that promotes balanced living and helps prompt the healing of autoimmune disorders and chronic illnesses"

—**Nick Nanton**, 15-time Emmy Award-Winning Producer/Director

MULTIDIMENSIONAL HEALING

A 12-Week Program to Reverse and Prevent Autoimmune Disorders and Other Chronic Illnesses

DR. TONI CAMACHO

BALBOA.PRESS
A DIVISION OF HAY HOUSE

Balboa Press books may be ordered through booksellers or by contacting:

Balboa Press
A Division of Hay House
1663 Liberty Drive
Bloomington, IN 47403
www.balboapress.com
844-682-1282

Print information available on the last page.

ISBN: 978-1-9822-1487-6 (sc)
ISBN: 978-1-9822-1488-3 (hc)
ISBN: 978-1-9822-1491-3 (e)

Library of Congress Control Number: 2018911620

Balboa Press rev. date: 06/06/2022

CONTENTS

ACKNOWLEDGMENTS

This work is dedicated with love and affection to my son, Daniel and to Gerhard, who inspired this book. Thank you both for your unconditional love and support and for believing in me.

Also with great gratitude, I'd like to acknowledge and thank the various teachers and mentors who have contributed to my knowledge and supported my development over the years, Seymour Koblin, Hugo Anguiano, John Finch, Jane Richmond, and Joe Guarino, amongst others.

Also thanks to the many others who had a significant impact on my development as well as inspired me in spirit through their books, seminars, and other work, Wayne Dyer, Jack Canfield, Pema Chodron, Dalai Lama, Rosemary Gladstar, and Louise Hay, to name but a few.

And finally thanks to my family, Mom, Dad, Ruben, Yideth, Santiago, Stacey, and all my friends, as well as those who assisted in making this effort a reality, Brenda De Hoyos-Aguilar, Melody Jones, Kallie Alderton, Denise Summey, and Fred Lalas.

INTRODUCTION

Macrobiotic living is the process of changing ourselves so that we can eat anything we like without the fear of becoming ill; it enables us to live a joyful life during which we can achieve anything we choose.

—GEORGE OSAWA

In this book, I'm going to share with you the key elements to health, well-being, and longevity. I am a nutritionist, holistic health practitioner, Reiki Master, and doctor of psychology. I am also a registered herbalist and have been professionally trained on how to design and make herbal medicine.

Throughout the last twenty years, I have studied health and spirituality under many different teachers and modalities. I have also taken many classes and seminars and read hundreds of books. Therefore, many schools of thoughts and mentors have influenced me. My training includes eastern and western nutrition, herbology, energy medicine, Shiatsu, and Tibetan Buddhist and Clinical psychology. This book is a short compilation of the concepts I have learned and applied successfully throughout these years, as well as the experience I have gained while working with many clients in clinic.

The concepts I'm sharing with you can help you heal from chronic illness as well as prevent disease, just as they have helped my family, friends, over a hundred of my clients, and even me. On December 2004, I was diagnosed with adrenal fatigue and post-traumatic stress disorder (PTSD). A lifetime of stress, anxiety, overwork, and neglecting my body had finally caught up with me. My condition was severe. The activity of my adrenal glands was so diminished that I had difficulty staying awake for more than a few hours per day.

My body was significantly affected, and I had many other symptoms, such as weakened immunity, sleep disturbances, and an inability to handle physical or emotional stress. I saw many doctors, and all told me that there was no solution for this condition.

Not being a person who is known for quitting easily, I decided to look for an answer in natural medicine. Therefore, I turned to the knowledge I acquired over the years and started applying concepts of natural medicine to my life, including nutrition, herbs, energy medicine, and personal counseling, amongst others.

Through my journey to health, I learned the importance of the mind-body connection, the power of compassion, and how the food we eat and the thoughts we think affects our physiology. This experience helped me find my life purpose and inspired me to share this knowledge with others. I know now that my purpose is to empower and support people on their journey to health, happiness, and self-love so they are free to focus on creating the life of their dreams.

My goal for this book is to provide a brief overview of the concepts I have found useful and effective for my clients and me and to guide you through a twelve-week program that will improve your quality of life immediately and get you started on your journey to health, happiness, and overall well-being.

This book is not intended to be a comprehensive study of nutrition, herbs, or psychotherapy. Instead it provides a brief overview of many concepts that you can use as a springboard to engage in these topics in detail in the future.

I believe the power to heal yourself is within you. All you must do is incorporate these health concepts into your life. You will see a recurring theme in this book, balance. I intend to make the idea of equilibrium hip again, making it a new fad. We are a society of excess and extremes, and it is for our health benefit that we relearn the old adage of moderation. Balance is one of the critical elements of health. Like Oscar Wilde said, "Everything in moderation, including moderation."

The majority of my work is based on the concepts of natural medicine, in particular, Eastern traditional medicine. In our society, traditional medicine is often referred to as alternative or holistic medicine. However, the World Health Organization (WHO) defines traditional medicine as "the sum total of the knowledge, skills, and practices based on the theories, beliefs, and experiences indigenous to different cultures, whether explicable or not, used in the maintenance of health as well as in the prevention, diagnosis, improvement or treatment of physical and mental illness".

However, I am a firm believer in science. Therefore, I will do my best to correlate the concepts of traditional medicine with the scientific research that validates it. You will find a lot of science in this book. Nevertheless, there are some traditional medicine concepts in this book that I found useful that science has not yet investigated.

At the same time, traditional medicine has been around for thousands of years, and even if we do not have the science to prove a specific component, we have millions of case studies that can validate that it works. Like one of my Chinese medicine teachers used to say, "Thousands of years of experience and millions of Chinese can't all be wrong."

In part one, I will cover why a holistic approach to health is the best approach for health and longevity. I will explain the mind-body connection and how your emotions impact your health. I will also discuss the first and second secret to health and how balanced living is essential to health. This means considering all aspects of your life: diet, relationships, work, fitness, environment, and emotional well-being. I will also cover basic herbal medicine concepts, teach you how to use herbs, and make the best of the medicinal herbs you have in your kitchen. I'm dedicating a significant portion of this section to basic nutritional concepts as well as an explanation of how the food you eat affects your emotional state. This is the most substantial part of this book. However, I feel it is necessary to have a good understanding of these concepts to understand why I designed this program the way I did.

In part two, I will explain why people get sick. Even though my intent for this book is to keep it as positive as possible, it is worth taking a little bit of time to go over in some detail the main factors that are the cause of chronic illness and autoimmune disorders. I promise to keep it short but informative so you can have a better understating on what may be making you sick, and if you are well, you can take the necessary measures to prevent illness.

Once you learn in part two what makes people sick and what steps you need to take to heal, part three will provide a list of principles that can improve your health. It will include recipes, exercises, and suggestions of techniques to help you heal your body or emotions.

Finally, in part four, I will take you on a step-by-step twelve-week program where you will apply the concepts you learned in part three. I am keeping the process as simple as possible. All you have to do is follow the steps listed for each week. This is where you put all that you learn in this book together, and then your life and health changes for the better.

PART ONE
Healing is Multidimensional

By means of personal experimentation and observation, we can discover certain simple and universal truths. The mind moves the body, and the body follows the mind. Logically then, negative thought patterns harm not only the mind but also the body. What we actually do builds up to affect the subconscious mind and in turn affects the conscious mind and all reactions.

—H. E. DAVEY, JAPANESE YOGA:
THE WAY OF DYNAMIC MEDITATION

CHAPTER ONE

Why a Multidimensional Approach to Health?

The doctor of the future will give no medicine, but will interest his patients in the care of the human frame, in diet, and in the cause and prevention of disease.

—THOMAS EDISON

A traditional holistic approach to health is multidimensional. It consists of medical aspects of traditional knowledge that developed over generations within various societies before the era of modern medicine. It emphasizes an equilibrium of the mind, body, and environment, and its focus is on health rather than disease. Furthermore, the emphasis is on the overall condition of the individual rather than on the particular illness or disease from which an individual is suffering, and the use of food and herbs is a core part of all holistic systems of medicine.[1]

Traditional medicine has successfully applied this multidimensional approach for centuries, and in the late twentieth century, science began to recognize the value of herbs, a proper diet, and the interaction between psychological processes and the nervous and immune systems. Now, not only is more and more research demonstrating the importance of herbs and diet to our health, it also shows how changes in human consciousness produce changes in the human body. This research reveals how our bodies respond to each of our thoughts and feelings and create cascades of biochemicals in our bodies and how each experience produces a positive or negative change in our cells.[2]

Likewise, science is showing us that genes determine physical characteristics such as eye color and height. However, our environment and consciousness—including our beliefs about health and aging, prayers, thoughts, intentions, and faith—contribute to our health, happiness, and longevity more than our genes. In fact, "Genes account for about 35% of longevity, while lifestyles, diet, and other environmental factors, including support systems, are the major reason people live longer," states Blair Justice, PhD, in his book, *Who Gets Sick*.[3]

This is clearly seen in identical twins when one develops a condition such as rheumatoid arthritis or cancer and the other does not. While identical twins share the same genes, researchers in epigenetics and gene expression are discovering that environmental factors influence how each of their genes is expressed.

Such is the case with Josephine Tesauro and her identical twin. At ninety-two, Josephine had a straight back and was vibrant and healthy. She lived alone and worked a part-time job in a hospital gift shop. Josephine drove herself to work, bridge clubs, church, and the grocery store.

On the other hand, her sister, at the same age, was incontinent. She had a hip replacement, suffered from a degenerative disorder that destroyed most of her vision, and had dementia. Josephine and her sister have identical genes, and yet they have completely different health paths. This seems to be a prevalent phenomenon observed in identical twins.

In his studies, Mario F. Fraga of the Spanish National Cancer Center has observed that, early in life, identical twins' genetic expression is indistinguishable. However, older sets of twins show significant differences in their gene expression and medical histories, and this is more noticeable in twins that have spent the most time apart,[4] leading scientists to conclude that lifestyle and the environmental factors play a significant role in the development of diseases.

Additionally research in epigenetics now shows us that genes only produce potentiality, a foundation, and not a specific phenomenon. According to Gary Marcus, PhD, it is more precise to think of genes as "providers of opportunities" or "sources of options" than "as rigid dictators of destiny."[5]

At the same time, researchers report that our thoughts, feelings, and external environments—such as social networks, food, and toxins—turn our genes on and off. (This is called "genetic expression.") Therefore, the science of epigenetics supports what traditional medicine has said for thousands of years: our actions, feelings, and environment contribute to our health status. We are not victims of our genes; instead the condition of our health is in our hands. For this reason, to prevent or to heal from an illness, it is necessary to create an environment that supports our health and healing processes. And this environment must include activities that encourage an equilibrium between and within our mind and body.

INTEGRATING WITH NATURE

Traditional medicine has long encouraged lifestyle practices that prevent disease and guide us to live long, healthy lives. In fact, Chinese doctors used to be paid to keep their clients healthy. If a client became ill, the doctor would not be paid until the patient's health returned. Their focus was on prevention, and the majority of healing traditions assert that the key to prevention and healing comes from awareness. The purpose of awareness is to quiet the body and mind, unify body and spirit, and find inner peace. They believe that a strong, bright spirit leads to improved health and increased longevity.

Additionally a fundamental view of traditional medicine is that a human is a part of nature. Humans are an intimate part of our environment, and we depend on it as much as we influence it. As a result, traditional medicine maintains that the microcosm of a person's health is reflective of the macrocosm of life and the universe. For this reason, traditional medicine is highly concerned with how the environment affects our health and urges us to live in accord with nature rather than try to adapt nature to us. The focus is on how to maintain harmony within the body and between it and the outside world, and emotions and lifestyle are also considered as contributory factors in health and disease. As a result, practitioners of traditional medicine believe the *first secret* to longevity is to flow with the rhythm of nature, and they encourage us to live each day fully and actively. This means living lives that are rich, full of experience, and without limits to our personal nature.

For this reason, from the perspective of traditional medicine, health can be defined this way: where there is movement and free flow, there's health. Likewise, blockages, stagnation, and fixation in the human body energy flow cause disease, or a lack of ease.

Many examples in nature reveal this principle. Such is the case with a stream. When a stream is flowing, it has clean water and sustains a healthy and plentiful ecosystem. In other words, the stream is considered healthy. However, if you add a dam to the same stream, stopping the flow, you start to see dirty water; the growth of fungi, algae, and bacteria; and a decline of life.

In the same way, this can be observed in a human body. For instance, if you were to tourniquet your knee, everything from the knee down would be stripped of nourishment. Your lower leg would not have access to the blood supply and nutrients. Therefore, the blockage, or stagnation, would cause a lack of ease or disease.

Another example is exposure to toxins. Chinese medicine places the liver in command of the proper flow of energy so, if the liver is overwhelmed with outside toxins and our own metabolic waste products, it cannot fulfill its role correctly, and stagnation (disease) will result.

Further, extreme or chronic emotions can also trigger energy stagnation. When you have negative experiences, you may form limiting beliefs about yourself and the world around you. This, in turn, restricts you from different aspects of yourself, consequently creating a kind of blockage or form of stagnation within your system.

So, to stay healthy, a person must regularly adapt to the changes going on inside and outside the body. If a person does not adjust, illness will manifest as a disharmony in the body. Food, herbs, acupuncture, tai chi, psychotherapy, meditation, qi gong, and all other types of energy medicine are methods to eliminate stagnation in the body and to stimulate the flow of energy to promote health.

In traditional medicine, the *second secret* to health and longevity is eating well, and food therapy (herbs are considered food) is regarded as the highest form of medicine. The theory is that the body will not live well or long without eating a balanced, varied, and healthy diet. And the diet should respond to the changing needs of a person's body. It must adjust to the needs of the person's body changing over time. Consequently traditional medicine's diets tend to be more complex than our modern Western diets. They focus on finding the proper balance according to each person's constitution and condition at a given time.

THE FIVE ELEMENTS: WHERE THERE IS NO FLOW, THERE IS DISEASE. WHERE THERE IS FLOW, THERE IS NO DISEASE

Traditional medicine, particularly Eastern medicine, is some of the oldest approaches to mind-body medicine. They are systems of health developed approximately four thousand years ago through observing the patterns found in nature.

Both Traditional Chinese Medicine (TCM) and Ayurvedic medicine of India teach that consciousness is energy manifested into five basic principles or elements: wood (air for Ayurvedic), fire, water, earth, and metal (ether for Ayurvedic). These are known as the five elements, five phases, or five transformations.

The five elements system is a comprehensive template that organizes all natural phenomena into five groups or patterns. It is important to remember that the elements are merely names or symbols used to describe five different types of energies in nature and our bodies. They are not the energy itself.

The five element theory is not the only way in which Eastern medicine described health and disease, but it is one of my favorite methods and one I have used successfully in my practice for many years. Therefore, I will be referencing it throughout this book.

According to Eastern medicine, just as in nature, our personal ecosystem contains all five elements. They represent our cosmic anatomy. Each element has a part to play to keep the ecosystem balanced, and they intertwine and balance one another to keep our bodies healthy. Disruption of one of the five element energies increases the risk of emotional disturbances or disruption in the pattern of flow of energy in our bodies. This may lead a person to experience specific ailments or emotions.

The five element system is a diagnostic tool that, along with other theories, can help us understand what is currently shaping our physical, mental, and spiritual health. To understand the five elements, we must first look at what each element compromises. Then we can examine what elements are dominant in our body and influencing our health. Each of the five groups includes categories such as a season, climate, internal organ, body tissue, emotion, an aspect of the soul, taste, color, and sound, amongst other things. Below is a chart[6] that shows some of the elemental correspondences and traits of each element:

	Water	Wood (Air)	Fire	Earth	Metal
Movement	Flowing	Rising	Radiating	Grounding	Gathering
Organs	Kidney Bladder	Liver Gallbladder	Heart Small intestine	Stomach Spleen Pancreas	Lungs Large intestine
Personality Traits	Openness Courage Flow	Direction Freshness Spontaneity	Excitement Variety	Nurturing Safety Compassion	Dependability Regularity
Natural Skill	Flexibility Adaptability	Creating new activity	Expansion Inspiration	Focus Carry through	Completing Moving on
Natural Challenge	Integrating change Flow	Loss of freedom	Focusing on one endeavor	Focus Carry through	Completing Moving on

	Water	Wood (Air)	Fire	Earth	Metal
Emotion When Out of Balance (Unhealthy)	Fear Insecurity Backing away	Anger when controlled Frustration Impatience Rage	Excitement Laughing Scattered Manic ups and downs Joy	Pity Suspicion Gossip Victim Blames others Abandoned Worry Anxiety	Sadness Guilt Depression Blames self Controlling Inferiority Shame Grief Melancholy
When Balanced (Healthy) Feeling	Adventurous Adaptable Go with the flow	Spontaneity Organization Patience Fresh	Radiant Inspiring Charismatic	Empathetic Supporting	Dependable Successful Complete
Relationship Strength	Seeing overall Big view Intuitive Awareness	Discovering Empowering New direction	Inspiring Passionate	Bonding Listening	Commitment Devotion
Relationship Weakness	Easily detached	Power quest	Multiple interests	Insecure Blaming others	Guilt Shame Being right or wrong
Tone of Voice	Apologetic Groaning Timid	Directing Shouting	Excited Verbose	Singing Whine	Monotone Choked
Emotive Response	Shivers	Gripping	Hyperactive Nervous	Sobbing Energy draining	Stuck Isolated Barren
Season	Winter	Spring	Summer	Early fall	Autumn
Body Association	Bones Head hair	Muscle Tendons Ligaments Nails	Blood vessels Face color Complexion	Interstitial fluid Lymph Breast Upper lip	Skin Breath Body hair
Body Fluids	Urine	Tears	Perspiration	Saliva	Mucus Snivel
Sense Organ	Hearing	Vision	Taste	Touch	Smell
Environment	Cold	Wind	Heat	Moisture	Dryness
Imbalanced Order	Putrefying Example: Urine	Oily Greasy Example: Rancid oil	Burning Scorched Example: Burned toast	Stale sweetness Example: Old perfume	Rancid Example: Fecal matter
Complexion Hue	Grayish	Dark brown Yellow Green	Red	Orangish Yellow	Sallow Pale white

	Water	Wood (Air)	Fire	Earth	Metal
Harmonizing Color	Dark shades Soothing rustic Blue Purple Black	Bright Fresh Pure Green	Inspiring yet grounding colors	Yellow Orange	White
Harmonizing Recommendations	Small challenges	Free play and recreation Avoid pressure Example: Competition	Focus One step at a time	Supportive environment Accept role as a participant	Variety Forgive
Harmonizing Taste	Salty	Sour	Bitter	Sweet	Pungent
Harmonizing Grains	Buckwheat Beans	Barley Wheat Rye	Corn Amaranth Quinoa	Millet	Rice
Harmonizing Vegetables	Seaweeds (cooked) Beans	Rising greens Example: Leeks, onions, celery, sprouts	Large, leafy greens Example: Kale, collards, dandelion	Round vegetables Example: Squash, pumpkin, cabbage, cauliflower	Contracted plants Roots Example: Radish, onion, burdock, carrot
Harmonizing Fruits	Winter and dried fruits	Spring fruits	Summer fruits	Late summer fruits	Autumn fruits

As previously mentioned, we can use these principles of natural law to help us heal and balance our bodies and emotions. By classifying your health difficulties within the above associations, we can look to see if a deficiency or excess of one of the elements in our body could be contributing to illness or emotional issue. For example, if a person complains about continually feeling cold, hearing problems, and frequent urination and has a dark complexion and timid attitude, this will lead us to conclude that the water element is out of balanced and possibly kidneys require attention.

BALANCING THE ELEMENTS

Eastern medicine physicians understand the cause and development of disease on the interrelated patterns of the five element theory. And it is believed that keeping all elements in balance promotes harmony both in our surroundings and ourselves. In this theory, each organ is either nourished or controlled by one of the others. As a result, disease could progress from one organ to another due to lack of nourishment, overcontrol, or abuse of an elemental energy. For example, if a person is in constant fear about the future, it is believed that he or she is overly expressing water (kidney) element energy, and with time, this will impact a different element, such as wood (liver). Consequently he or she will experience wood energy symptoms too, such as anger or frustration.

According to this system, each element acts upon two others, either giving birth to it or controlling it. For example, wood gives birth to fire and controls or suppresses earth. Likewise, fire gives birth to earth and controls metal. All the elements are continually interacting with other elements. None stands alone. The table below (figure 1) outlines the relationships.

Element Gives Birth To	Element Controls
Wood - Fire	Wood - Earth
Fire - Earth	Earth - Water
Earth - Metal	Water – Fire
Metal - Water	Fire – Metal

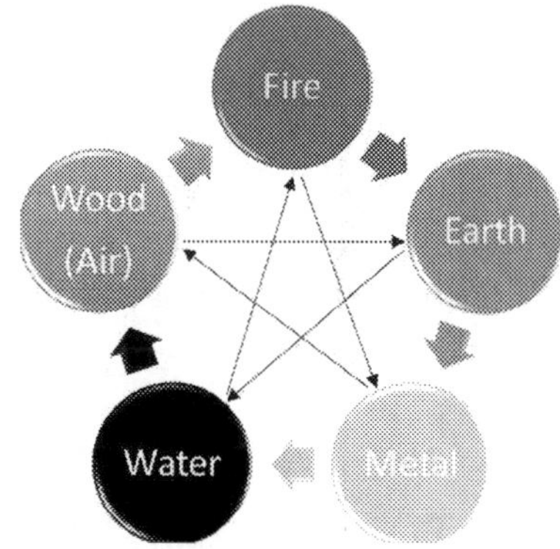

Figure. 1—Five element generating sequence or cycle.

Therefore, treatment of a deficient or malfunctioning body organ was often based on strengthening the organ corresponding to the element preceding it in the cycle, minimizing the energy of the element that is controlling it or bringing more energy of the element that is deficient. Which approach to use will depend on the condition of the person. For instance, to resolve a kidney (water) imbalance, we can minimize earth energy in our lives by taking responsibility for our lives instead of blaming others, or we can bring more of the water element by eating more warm soups and seaweed to balance the excess cold in our bodies.

A detailed look at the use of five element theory to diagnosing and treating illnesses is beyond the scope of this book. However, I took the time to describe this theory because it is one of the methods that this health program is based on and I will be referencing this theory throughout the rest of the book.

THE BEST APPROACH TO HEALTH AND LONGEVITY IS MULTIDIMENSIONAL

As previously mentioned, the connection among the mind, body, and environment has been a central theme in many healing traditions for thousands of years. And a large part of the population in developing countries still rely on traditional practitioners and herbs for their primary care. However, during the past two decades, interest in natural therapies has increased tremendously in industrialized countries.[1]

This multidimensional approach to health is growing around the world and is used for promoting health as well as for preventing and curing diseases. Traditional medicine views human bodies as wholes, more than just a sum of parts. On the other hand, Western (conventional) medicine is reductionist. Therefore, it is full of specialists, focused on one organ or system of the body. However, the systems and organs of the human body do not work in isolation, and they are composed of many biochemical and bioenergetic feedback loops that cannot be looked at separately.

Moreover, approximately 60 percent of the causes of health problems and chronic illness cannot be explained by what conventional medicine often considers triggers, for example, pathogens, genetic factors, and so on. Consequently conventional medicine does not have an explanation for them,[7] and it reinforces the "treat symptoms" approach to health.

Additionally blood tests and other diagnostic techniques used by Western medicine to diagnose certain diseases are based on what conventional medicine calls "normal" ranges, but what happens when a person is experiencing symptoms but his or her numbers do not fall out of normal range? In most cases, you are told you are healthy, and it is the end of the story. And in worst scenarios, you are told it is all in your head.

Consequently this leaves people not only feeling ill but also frustrated, scared, and hopeless. This scenario is a common occurrence.

I have both experienced and heard this story from a countless number of clients. Our bodies and our environments are too complex to continue using this approach to health, which is why Western medicine is no longer serving us in cases of complex, out-of-the-box disorders such as autoimmune and chronic illnesses.

To heal means "to make whole." Therefore, when treating any disorder, it is important to treat the person and not the lab results because every illness or symptom is just a façade that hides or distracts us from the whole person. Therefore, we need to get through the layers of symptoms until the root of the problem gets addressed.

Consider the case of my client, Alice, who suffered from chronic candida for over twenty years. It was not until she approached her condition from different dimensions, in other words, taking into account, mind, body, and spirit, that she finally healed. This is her story.

> I went through much of my life thinking I was "healthy," but there were always nagging little issues that didn't hit the radar of conventional medicine. My blood tests were great. I was physically fit, mentally stable, and thin. I ate "healthy." I was a top-performing student. No issues, right? Not if you were me.
>
> Starting at age ten or eleven, I had chilblains. It's something more likely to be found in the cold damp of the United Kingdom than San Diego. It's an excruciating condition resulting from circulation issues. Conventional medical doctors had heard of it but never seen it. Then I started having recurring yeast infections and split lips beginning in high school and continuing through my thirties. Short menstrual cycles and painful cramps were just part of life until I finally insisted on not living in pain and trying to understand the source of things. I started acupuncture and went on an anti-candida diet in 2007: gluten-free, no sugar, no fruit, no alcohol, and so forth. It was better, but it wasn't enough. I still had symptoms if I strayed even just a little.

Add to the above, working long hours under somewhat stressful circumstances in my thirties, I started getting fatigued, emotionally volatile, and brain fog. (I couldn't remember conversations, wasn't as analytically sharp, and so on.) At that point, I decided enough was enough and started to try to treat what I found out was candida overgrowth through diet. It was an extremely restrictive diet. I had tried Diflucan and various over-the-counter drugs and found out I was only treating symptoms, not the cause. I also found out that candida is primarily due to an imbalance in gut flora caused by antibiotics. I had had numerous rounds of antibiotics as a preteen and teen for two different mouth surgeries and various ensuring complications and possibly other times that I don't remember. Then in my late thirties, I got hit with Ramsay Hunt syndrome, paralysis in the face due to inflammation of the seventh cranial nerve, the final wake-up call. Once again, conventional medicine had rarely seen any cases. There was no real treatment other than a protocol for Bell's palsy and few doctors with any real knowledge. I had to change my lifestyle even further—reduce stress at work and so forth.

By now, I was in my early forties. Yeast infections were managed, but not gone. I found out through numerous tests and a fantastic doctor that my candida was a symptom of more significant issues—hormone imbalance, parasites, and heavy metal toxicity. The aha moment. My body was under extreme stress. I treated the parasites, chelated the heavy metals, and balanced the hormones, but still continued to have issues with yeast. Twenty-five-plus years of candida buildup isn't easy to get rid of or treat.

Enter Dr. Camacho. Dr. Toni helped eliminate the yeast imbalance (altogether verified through lab testing), balance my hormones, and help my circulation. It was not overnight, but over time as one issue was addressed, we could move on to others with very noticeable results. All of those years of stress on the body took a toll, so the treatment took six to nine months, but it worked. I now have more balanced gut flora. I've made permanent diet and lifestyle changes and have a firm belief that traditional medicine, emotional well-being, and spirituality have a lot to contribute to our overall health.

As you can see from Alice's case study, when it comes to health, there is more than just the body involved. By following a holistic perspective, I consider all dimensions that play a part in promoting health, not just the mechanics of the physical body.

The benefits of holistic medicine are vast. Nevertheless, the most common reasons for using traditional medicine are:

- Side effects from medical interventions, including medications, are avoided. Iatrogenic medicine (errors in medicine) is now the number-three leading cause of death in America.[8] And there is evidence pointing out that it may be the number-one leading cause of death.[9]
- Traditional medicine aims to correct the root cause(s) of an imbalance instead of solely focusing on resolving symptoms.
- Because the practitioner will consider the psychosocial, spiritual, and mental states that are causing the imbalance, the client will not only be making improvements toward his or her original health problem but also in many other areas of his or her life.
- Traditional medicine is more affordable.
- Traditional medicines, in general, are natural, safe, and nontoxic.
- Traditional medicine is a personalized health-care system. As a result, a client feels cared for.
- Traditional medicine has been shown to be a useful therapy option for chronic illnesses and in cases when conventional medicine is ineffective, such as in advanced cancer, autoimmune disorders, and new infectious diseases.

Besides, human physiology and the root of chronic illness has not changed. Therefore, even though traditional medicine is thousands of years old, it has not become obsolete. Moreover, a procedure is not invalid just because we do not have a scientific study to prove it works. There are hundreds of successful medical procedures that were discovered years before we had the studies to demonstrate the principles behind the treatment.

For example, we were using penicillin and aspirin before we understood their mechanisms of action, but we used them because we knew they worked. Some traditional medicine procedures and practices have been used successfully for thousands of years. That is why it is so crucial to our health system to remember root and origins of medicine, which is traditional medicine, even if science at this moment does not have a clear understanding of how some of the standard practices of traditional medicine work.

To conclude, traditional medicine encompasses a range of practices that promote equilibrium and bring us into a state of balance, but the core disciplines include herbalism, nutrition, energy medicine, and emotional healing. It is my opinion that, regardless of modality, a complete holistic healing system is a model of life-affirming principles that is highly adaptable to each individual and must give as much attention to the mind as the body. It is a comprehensive plan that incorporates moral and spiritual practices, lifestyle guidelines, and nutrition. For this reason, this system should feature at least the following components: herbal supplements, nutrition, activity (exercise), energy medicine, emotional healing (promote awareness), and possible changes to the internal and external environment.

The next section explores each one of these components in more detail.

CHAPTER TWO

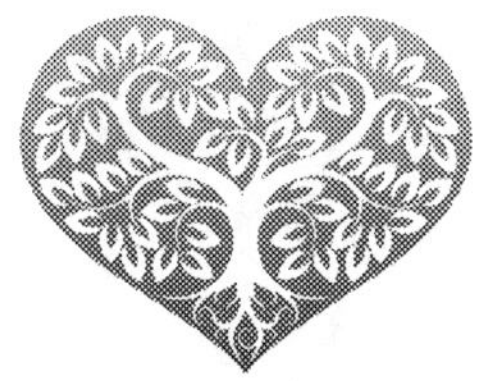

More on the Mind/Body Connection

We are shaped by our thoughts; we become what we think. When the mind is pure, joy follows like a shadow that never leaves.

—BUDDHA

As previously mentioned, in many traditional medicine modalities, the priority in the healing process is emotional health, and emotional health starts with mindful awareness. By learning to quiet the mind, awareness can free us from obstructed emotions. The focused, self-reflected mind is calm and clear. It observes with wisdom and strengthens the spirit. And a strong spirit leads to health and healing against any disease. Not to mention, when our emotions are in balance and we have self-love and self-respect, we naturally make quality choices of food and lifestyle that benefit our health.

The critical role that emotions play in healing and overall health cannot be overemphasized. According to Dr. Bernie Siegel, "We participate and are responsible for a lot of the things that happen to us." He states,

> If you hate your job, you are much more likely to get sick and die at a younger age than someone who's happy at work and has a nice family life and is mentally well adjusted. The mind and body are not separate units, but one integrated system. How we act and what we think, eat, and feel are all related to our health.

In fact, the latest scientific discoveries now classify unforgiveness as a disease. According to Dr. Steven Standiford, chief of surgery at the Cancer Treatment Centers of America, refusing to forgive makes people sick and keeps them ill. As a result, forgiveness therapy is now being used to help treat diseases, such as cancer. Dr. Standiford explains, "It's important to treat emotional wounds or disorders because they really can hinder someone's reactions to the treatments, even someone's willingness to pursue treatment."

In the same way, studies have found that the act of forgiveness can improve your health by lowering your risk of heart attack, improving your cholesterol levels and sleep, and reducing pain, blood pressure, anxiety, depression, and stress.

Moreover, according to research by Dr. Michael Barry, harboring the negative emotions associated with unforgiveness, such as anger and hatred, creates a state of chronic anxiety. He further states, "Chronic anxiety very predictably produces excess adrenaline and cortisol, which deplete the production of natural killer cells, which is your body's foot soldier in the fight against cancer."[10]

Besides, health and wellness are more than the absence of disease. The emerging concept of positive health focuses on promoting people's positive health assets, that is, strengths that can contribute to a healthier, happier, responsible, and longer life. These assets may not only include biological factors, such as high heart rate variability, but it will also include environmental factors, such as a stable marriage, and subjective factors, such as positive emotions like optimism and gratitude[10].

THE SCIENCE BEHIND THE POWER OF POSITIVE EMOTIONS.

H. E. Davey stated,

> Because all actions and expressions stem from the mind, it is vital to know the mind as well as decide in what way we'll use it. Everyone has heard of psychosomatic illness, and most of us acknowledge that psychosomatic sicknesses can and do occur. But what about psychosomatic wellness?

The connection between the mind and body is a central feature in many healing traditions. These traditions have long stressed the importance of positive emotions for our well-being. However, it is only recently that researchers have found out just how positive emotions such as happiness, compassion, engagement, purpose, positive accomplishments, and optimism protect from physical illness, and they also predict lack of depression, higher achievement, and physical health. Not only are these feelings profoundly healing and soothing, they also help people face the many challenges that may come their way.[11]

The following section illustrates some of the health benefits of these positive emotions, and in part three of this book, we will explore how to bring these emotions into our lives.

1. **Happiness.** "Real happiness starts when you begin to cherish others," said Lama Zopa Rinpoche. Our pursuit of meaning, justice, and happiness is as much a part of us today as it was centuries ago when humans could first give thought to these concepts. From the perspective of spiritual traditions, happiness involves a moral or spiritual relationship between the self, one's actions, and the Divine. Philosophers such as Aristotle, Plato, Aquinas, Buddha, and Confucius believed that virtues led to happiness. In fact, they considered virtue as the most essential component of happiness.[12] In his writings, Aristotle (VII.1323b1) states,

   > Happiness, whether consisting in pleasure or virtue, or both, is more often found with those who are highly cultivated in their minds and in their character and have only a moderate share of

external goods, than among those who possess external goods to a useless extent but are deficient in higher qualities.

The happiness these philosophers spoke of was not necessarily the same that we would think of today. For them, a happy individual exhibits a personality appropriately balanced between reasons and desires, with moderation characterizing all. A good life is one where an individual develops his or her strengths, realizes his or her potential, and becomes what it is in his or her nature to become, in other words, his or her life purpose.[13] They argued that pleasure is not good in itself since it is, by its nature, incomplete; however, worthwhile activities are often associated with their distinctive pleasures. Genuine happiness lies in action that leads to virtue since this alone provides real value and not just amusement. In this sense, virtue is its own reward. True happiness can therefore be attained only through the cultivation of virtues that make a human life complete[12] such as kindness, compassion, social intelligence, humor, courage, integrity, and the like. As a result, real happiness is defined by the measurement of life satisfaction and has three aspects: positive emotion, engagement, and meaning, each of which feeds into life satisfaction.

Besides, happiness and health are connected, and plenty of research supports that one's level of happiness is directly correlated with the level of one's health. The list below shows some of a few critical findings on the relationship between happiness and health.

- Cheerful people live longer.[14] In a longitudinal study, 90 percent of cheerful people were found to be alive at age eighty-five, whereas 34 percent of the unhappy people were alive at that age. Similarly, 54 percent of the happy people were alive at age ninety-four, while only 11 percent of the unhappy people were alive.
- Cheerful people have more marital satisfaction.[15]
- Happy people have lower blood pressure, and their immune system is more resistant.[15]
- Happy people are healthier, more prosperous, and more socially engaged.[16]

- There is plenty of evidence that chronic unhappiness such as depression, anxiety, and stress are linked to poor health. Studies show that these emotions can negatively affect immunity and increase inflammation in the body, leading to diseases.
- Happy people have a better outlook on life. Therefore, they are more prepared to handle tasks and any issues that come their way at any given time.[17]

2. **Optimism—Attitude Can Affect Your Health.** "A pessimist sees the difficulty in every opportunity; an optimist sees the opportunity in every difficulty," said Winston Churchill. Optimism can be defined as reacting to problems with a sense of confidence and high personal ability. In particular, optimistic individuals believe that adverse events are temporary, limited in scope, and manageable. Positive thinking and being optimistic is not just something that we do to help achieve our goals or to get through difficult times. Research has shown that a positive attitude has a significant effect on our health. Optimism has been proven to boost the immune system and prevent chronic illness. In fact, a positive attitude can add years to your lives. The following studies illustrate this:

   - Compared to pessimist people, people with high levels of optimism have a 50 percent lower risk of death from cardiovascular disease.[18]
   - Optimistic, happy people tend to die of old age, and less than 1 percent of these people tend to die of cancer or heart disease. On the other hand, 75 percent of people that die of heart disease and 15 percent of those who die of cancer are people with lifelong patterns of anger.[19]
   - People with a lifelong habit of hopelessness tend to die thirty-five years younger than self-actualized positive people do. 75 percent of them die of cancer, and 15 percent die of heart disease.[19]
   - Studies have shown that breast cancer survivors have much shorter survival times if they have a hopeless or helpless attitude.[20, 21]
   - Optimistic people have better memories and overall stay healthier.[22]

- There are much higher rates of depression in pessimistic people than optimists.[15]
- People with positive attitudes, in particular, beliefs about aging, were found to live seven and a half years longer than negative people do.[22]

3. **Practicing Gratitude Improves Emotional and Physical Well-being.** "Gratitude unlocks the fullness of life. It turns what we have into enough, and more. It turns denial into acceptance, chaos to order, confusion to clarity. It can turn a meal into a feast, a house into a home, a stranger into a friend," said Melody Beattie. "The practice of gratitude can have dramatic and lasting effects in a person's life," commented Robert A. Emmons, a leading scientific expert on the science of gratitude at UC Davis. Gratitude is associated with optimism, and studies have discovered that grateful people are happier, less stressed, and less depressed and receive more social support. Emmons believes gratitude allows individuals to celebrate the present and be an active participant in their own lives. By focusing on valuing and appreciating friends, oneself, situations, and circumstances, it focuses the mind of an individual on what he or she already has rather than something that's missing and is needed.

More on Gratitude Research

Gratitude is associated with higher levels of good cholesterol (HDL) and lower levels of bad cholesterol (LDL). People who write in a gratitude journal for fifteen minutes before they go to bed sleep better and longer.[23] Grateful people experience fewer aches and pains, lower blood pressure (even when under stress), and improved mental clarity, and they report feeling healthier than other people do.[24] Robert Emmons has concluded that gratitude improves psychological health such as increasing happiness and reducing depression. It also reduces toxic emotions, such as envy, resentment, frustration, and regret. Additionally, gratitude enhances empathy, reduces aggression, and improves self-esteem.

Gratitude increases mental strength and resilience, reduces stress, and helps to overcome trauma.[25, 26] Practicing gratitude led to a 7 percent reduction in biomarkers of inflammation in patients with congestive heart failure.[27] Keeping a gratitude diary for two weeks produced sustained reductions in perceived stress by 28 percent and depression by 16 percent.[28]

Gratitude lower levels of cortisol (stress hormones) by 23 percent. A daily gratitude practice can decrease the effects of neurodegeneration that occurs with increasing age. Writing a letter of gratitude reduced feelings of hopelessness in 88 percent of suicidal inpatients and increased levels of optimism in 94 percent. Grateful people have between 9 to 13 percent lower levels of Hemoglobin A1c, a key marker of glucose control that plays a vital role in diabetes.[29]

According to Cicero (106–43 BC), gratitude is not only the greatest of the virtues but the parent of all of the others. You will be surprised how the simple act of gratitude can change your life for the better. Not only will it improve your health, it will also lift your vibration and bring you into harmony with the energy of the universe, which in turn will attract more good things into your life to be grateful for.

4. **The Health Benefits of Love.** There is also evidence that many health benefits are gained from being involved in healthy relationships. Human beings are profoundly social animals who spend a large part of their time observing others and trying to understand what they are doing and why.[30] We are born to form attachments. "Our brains are physically wired to develop in tandem with another's through emotional communication, beginning before words are spoken."[31] Thus, one of the most important influences on well-being are social relationships, and when humans develop good relationships, the impact on our health is far-reaching. However, I am not talking about falling in love or romance. In fact, "There's no evidence that the intense, passionate stage of a new romance is beneficial to health," says Harry Reis, PhD, co-editor of the *Encyclopedia of Human Relationships*. "People who fall in love say it feels wonderful and agonizing at the same time." The ups and downs involved with falling in love can be a source of

stress. Instead, "It takes a calmer, more stable form of love to yield clear health benefits."

"There is very nice evidence that people who participate in satisfying, long-term relationships fare better on a whole variety of health measures." The key is to "feel connected to other people, feel respected and valued by other people, and feel a sense of belonging," she says. Here are research-backed ways that love impact our health:

- Individuals in healthy, committed relationships have fewer doctor's visits and shorter hospital stays.
- Getting married or being in a committed relationship reduces depression (if either is healthy).
- A healthy, committed relationship contributes to a decline in heavy drinking and drug abuse.
- People in a healthy, committed relationship have the lowest blood pressure, followed by single people with a strong social connection. On the other hand, unhappily married people have the worst blood pressure numbers.
- People in healthy, long-term relationships have a more active dopamine-reward area. Consequently they have less anxiety.
- Long-term couples show more activity in the parts of the brain that manages pain.
- People who have the support of someone who loves them are better to cope with stressful situations.
- Loving, healthy relationships boost the immune system. Therefore, they are less likely to get sick after being exposed to a cold or flu virus.
- The wounds of people in happy, positive relationships heal twice as fast compared with couples who have negative feelings toward each other.
- People in a happily, committed relationship live longer.

- People in healthy relationships with a partner or family are happier.

Even though the majority of these studies were done with couples in committed relationships, Reis believes this is not only true for romantic partnerships. The effects extend to other close relationships such as a parent, child, or friend. For example, other studies have shown:

- Love minimizes the effects of stress and eases anxiety. "Just being in the presence of someone who greets us with positive regard and caring can actually lower those levels of cortisol and adrenaline and create greater homeostasis, which means that your neurochemicals are back in balance," says Reis.
- Touch can ease pain, lift depression, and even increase the odds that a team will win.
- Babies who are not held and hugged enough will stop growing. And if the situation lasts long enough, even if they are receiving proper nutrition, they die.

Likewise, according to psychology professor Ed Diener, family and friends are crucial for well-being, and the wider and deeper the relationships with those around you, the better.[32] In addition to Diener, the Dalai Lama also recommends maintaining closeness with as many people as possible in order to live a happy life.[33] A human's need for people is paradoxical, he states. "While their culture is caught up in the celebration of fierce independence, they also yearn for intimacy and connection with a special loved one."[34]

Moreover, without human friendship, an individual's life becomes miserable, and yet humans are used to feeling like separate individuals. Consequently they are less likely to pay much attention to the fact that their everyday experience is a shared reality,[35] as Einstein notes,

> A human being is part of a whole, called by us the Universe, a part limited in time and space. He experiences himself, his thoughts and feelings, as something separated from the rest a kind of optical delusion of his consciousness. This delusion is a kind of prison for us, restricting us to our personal desires and to affection for a few

> persons nearest us. Our task must be to free ourselves from this prison by widening our circles of compassion to embrace all living creatures and the whole of nature in its beauty. Nobody is able to achieve this completely, but the striving for such achievement is in itself a part of the liberation and a foundation for inner security.

Thus, we are designed to be emotionally entangled. As Einstein expressed, our deepest human nature is essentially interdependent. All beings and phenomena are caused to exist by other beings and phenomena (Buddha Net, 1996–2011), and each individual has a role to play in sustaining the whole.[35]

Furthermore, Dr. Keltner from UC Berkley also points out that we are interconnected. "It is in our DNA, we are born to be our brother's keeper."[36] It is our capacity to be profoundly moved by each other that makes us whole. There is no such thing as a separate feeling, breath, or emotion. Everything has an impact. According to biologist Juan Manuel Carrion, everything in nature has a purpose and no single purpose is more important than another.

> There is a great lesson I learned from nature, from the birds, the insects, from the ecosystems: The awareness that everything has its reason to exist in nature, nothing is redundant; nothing insignificant. A spider is as important as a dragonfly, an insect, a bird, a mammal, or a huge tree. Perhaps a tiny plant has a specific and important function that makes it as important as a giant tree. This is the awareness that everything has its purpose, and nothing is insignificant because everything has its own value.
>
> Therefore, we are born to be in community, and no one is born free from the need for love and connectedness. Thus, how we live with and relate to each other and the earth matters, what we do at an individual level affects others, and despite the fact that the process of relating to others might involve hardships and quarrels, individuals have to keep an attitude of friendship and warmth in order to lead a way of life in which there is enough interaction with other people to enjoy a happy and healthy life.[33]

5. **The Effects of Compassion and Altruism on Health.** Altruism and compassion also have health-promoting effects on the immune system and autonomic nervous system as well as cardiovascular efficiency. They also reduce the secretion of the stress hormone cortisol. Therefore, they can protect us from physical illness. Research has proven that, when we fantasize and think about compassion, it stimulates areas of our brain and body in ways that are beneficial to our health and well-being. Compassion or good feelings toward others release oxytocin, endorphins, and other biochemicals in the brain that generate feelings of warmth, euphoria, and connection to others. These good feelings are reflected in our biology. Therefore, not only can doing good can make people feel good, it also improves their overall well-being.

   There are significant health benefits to compassion, volunteerism, and giving:

   - Giving produces endorphins in the brain that provide a mild version of morphine high.[37]
   - Oxytocin causes people to give more and feel more empathy toward others, even if we do not see or experience the positive effects of our gifts.[38]
   - People who practice compassion produce 100 percent more DHEA, a hormone that counteracts the aging process, and 23 percent less cortisol, the stress hormone.[39]
   - Those who gave contributions of time or money are 42 percent more likely to be happy than those who do not donate.[40]
   - When individuals perform altruistic acts, they activate regions of the brain associated with pleasure (like food or sex), social connection, and trust, creating a warm glow effect they call "helper's high."[37]
   - Donating affects two brain reward systems that are also stimulated by food, sex, drugs, and money and an area of the brain that is related to social attachments.[41]

- Rejecting certain causes stimulates the lateral orbitofrontal cortex (LOFC), which is linked to anger, moral disgust, and other aversive traits.[41]
- Meditation of loving-kindness and compassion are associated with feelings of happiness.[42]
- Meditation on compassion seems to strengthen connections and functioning in the parts of the brain that calm such feelings as fear or anger.[42]
- Cultivating compassion and kindness through meditation affects brain regions that can make a person more empathic to other peoples' mental states.[43]
- People feel good when focusing on another, which can reduce preexisting distress. In other words, a positive mood can result from being other-focused.[17]

6. **Spirituality—The Power of Belief.** Last but not least, a growing body of research indicates that spirituality, religion, and prayer play an important role in health and wellness. Feeling you are part of something greater than yourself makes you feel happier, grateful, and grounded, with purpose and hopefully an awareness of your own uniqueness in the universe. Studies show that people that consider themselves spiritual regardless of religion or spiritual practice are more likely to:

- report being very happy[44]
- have a longer life[45]
- have a lower risk of depression[46] and suicide[47]
- be more resilient (be better able to cope with illness, depression, and stress)
- be more faithful in relationships[48]
- have happier children[48] and be more satisfied with their family life[49]

- have lower psychological distress, sleep disturbance, and fatigue[50]
- have a better quality of life if you have cancer or other chronic illness[50]

Likewise, we can use the power of belief and visualization to heal. Our minds have the ability to change our chemistry and consequently help us recover from illness. It works in the same way an athlete uses visualization to improve performance, says Dr. Bernie Siegel. We have seen this in many case studies, like in the case of Oscar winner for original screenplay David Seidler.

Seidler, at seventy-three, suffered and survived cancer, and he says he did so by visualizing his cancer away. "I know it sounds awfully Southern California and woo-woo," he admits, "but that's what happened." When Seidler found out his cancer had returned, he visualized a "lovely, clean healthy bladder" for two weeks, and afterward the cancer was gone.

CONNECTING THE DOTS BETWEEN PHYSICAL HEALTH AND EMOTIONS

In conclusion, all the studies reviewed reinforce that positive emotions, thoughts, and prayers play an essential role in an individual's health and overall well-being. Science has proven what spiritual traditions, such as Buddhism, have stated for thousands of years. Unhappy or stressed-out thoughts are a contributing factor to poor health and lack of overall well-being. Therefore, to be truly healthy, it is equally as important to take the time and effort to nurture both your body and your emotions.

For this reason alone, why not consider making a daily habit to perform activities that boost your positive emotions, such as meditation, breathing exercises, gratitude journaling, volunteer work, and so on. It would be worth it, right?

CHAPTER THREE

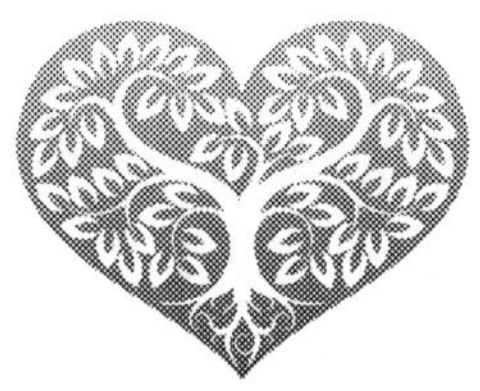

The Role of Nutrition in Health

When diet is wrong, medicine is of no use. When diet is correct, medicine is of no need.

—AYURVEDIC PROVERB

As previously mentioned, the role of proper nutrition in health is vital, so much that and in traditional medicine, the second secret to health and longevity is eating well. Food is an essential part of life. The consumption of food and liquid gives us energy and the necessary nutrients to sustain life and to meet our body's basic needs for growth, development, and function. Without proper nutrition, our bodies are more prone to disease, infection, fatigue, and poor performance.

More importantly, every cell in the body depends on the right quantity (balance) and continuous supply of the following five nutrients from the food we eat to stay healthy and productive:

- Proteins are needed to build, maintain, and repair muscle, blood, skin, bones, and other tissues and organs in the body.
- Carbohydrates provide the body with its primary source of energy. Carbohydrates can be classified into two kinds: starches and sugars.
- Fats (good fats) are the body's secondary source of energy and provide more energy/calories per gram than any other nutrient; so they are difficult to burn.
- Vitamins and minerals are needed in small amounts but are essential for good health. They control many functions and processes in the body, and in the case of minerals, they also help build body tissue such as bones (calcium) and blood (iron).

Proper nutrition is essential for achieving optimal health because our organs and tissues need adequate nutrition to work effectively. Moreover, *extreme diets* that emphasize eating one type of nutrient over another might help you lose weight, but in the long run, they set you up for life-threatening medical conditions. Because so many foods are excluded from these diets, they are unbalanced and not recommended. For example, eliminating beans, legumes, and whole grains from your diet may leave you low in fiber, B vitamins, and minerals like magnesium and selenium. Overeating saturated fats like butter and large amounts of red meat increase the amount of cholesterol in your blood, thereby multiplying your risk of developing heart disease. Overeating protein can also hurt your body. Over thirty years of research studies concur that long-term excess protein consumption has been linked to osteoporosis and kidney disease.[51, 52]

In fact, this is what happens to your body when you don't eat carbs, drink every meal, or deprive your body of the calories it needs. You become dehydrated and create blood sugar imbalances. Your muscles break down, and your metabolism slows down. Malnutrition begins. Your brain suffers.

Therefore, before eliminating a particular food or food group from your diet, try instead eating it in the appropriate quantity and in a high-quality form (unless you are allergic to them). For example, instead of avoiding rice, eat organic brown rice that has been soaked overnight before being cooked. I will cover more on the topic of how to eat later in this chapter.

THE ELEMENTS OF BASIC NUTRITION

It is essential that the food you eat is as close as its natural state as it can be. These are known as *whole foods*. A whole food is intact and in its natural state. It has not been processed or refined. Therefore, it contains all the vitamins, minerals, and other nutrients that are part of the food. Whole foods have many benefits, such as keeping your immune system healthy and preventing disease.

Additionally, your nutritional needs should be met primarily through your diet. Supplements are not meant to replace a healthy diet, and taking too much of certain vitamins or minerals in the long run can harm you. Therefore, it is recommended to first make an effort to improve your diet and lifestyle before you supplement. If you are unable to make dietary or lifestyle changes, you have a deficiency in a nutrient, or you are weak, then use supplements.

The reason is that nutrients are the most potent when they come from food. When scientists have attempted to isolate single components from foods and incorporate them into a pill for disease prevention, studies suggest that these molecules in their isolated form do not offer the same gains as when they are eaten from whole food sources.

For example, eating fruits and vegetables high in antioxidants reduces the risk for cardiovascular disease, certain types of cancer, memory loss, and progressive eye diseases. However, taking a specific antioxidant has failed to show that supplemental antioxidants significantly decrease the risk of the health conditions previously mentioned.

WHY EAT ORGANIC OR WILDCRAFTED?

Growers judge the quality of a plant by its mineral content. With better mineralization, more significant quantities of vitamins and phytonutrients are found in the plant. Quite a few reliable studies indicate that organic foods have substantially more minerals, as much as 90 percent more compared with nonorganic foods. These studies suggest that organic foods provide us with better nutrition.

Moreover, studies have demonstrated that glyphosate, an active ingredient in herbicides (pesticides), is the most important causal factor in the development of gluten intolerance. A characteristic of gluten intolerance is the impairment in many cytochrome P450 enzymes, which are needed to detoxify environmental toxins, activate vitamin D3, catabolize vitamin A, and maintain bile acid production and sulfate supplies to the gut. Not to mention glyphosate is known to cause gut bacteria imbalance; deficiencies in iron, cobalt, molybdenum, copper, and other rare metals; and deficiencies in tryptophan, tyrosine, methionine, and selenomethionine.

Gluten intolerance and gut imbalance have a significant impact to people's health. For example, gluten-intolerant people have an increased risk of non-Hodgkin's lymphoma and reproductive issues such as infertility, miscarriages, and birth defects. All of this can also be linked to glyphosate exposure.[53]

Additionally, practically all meat in the United States that is not organic is produced using one or more hormones. Hormones are used to accelerate the growth of animals, consequently speeding production and reducing costs. Some scientists believe there is a potential for these types of hormones to cause reproductive and metabolic problems in humans. Also hydrolyzed proteins that contain MSG are now being introduced to lean cuts of meat to add flavor and tenderize them.

Likewise, for the past forty-plus plus years, the beef industry has been continually administering low levels of antibiotics to compensate for the conditions that exist in overcrowded feedlots. Otherwise sickness could spread fast and eradicate the entire herd. This overuse of antibiotics has led to antibiotic resistance in animals and humans. Experts have raised concerns about farm-raised fish too, which in some cases are also raised on unnatural diets and crammed into small enclosures that can breed disease, promoting heavily on antibiotics.

On the other hand, research has found that dairy products and meat from grass-fed cattle can have CLA levels at 30 percent to 50 percent higher than those of animals fed a diet of primarily corn and grain. CLA is a trans-fatty acid that is healthy and has been shown to contain both antioxidant and anticancer properties.

It is important to note that certified organic meats come from animals that are not allowed to eat food that has been treated with synthetic fertilizers, pesticides, herbicides, or radiation. Their food sources cannot contain any preservatives, additives, or GMOs.

Furthermost, most of the nonorganic food in the US is genetically modified. The topic of genetic engineering (GE) of our food is one that is highly charged with political and economic issues and is not the intention of this book to go into any of them. Instead I will focus on the GE effects on nutrition.

The GE of food involves the transfer of genes into seeds from different species, such as animals (including humans), fish, insects, bacteria, viruses, and other plants to improve the crop. Gene alterations, which is not a precisely controlled process, often disrupts the DNA sequence in an organism. These new genes change cell chemistry and provoke toxins and allergens that the human body has not experienced before.[54]

More importantly, plants are being genetically engineered and sold before the risk has been thoroughly assessed.[54] Reason being, unlike drugs that are designed to cause a change in the human bodies, GMOs are created to be equivalent to their non-GE counterparts. Therefore, scientists do not see a mechanism of harm in GMOs, and without a reasonable mechanism whereby injury may occur, how can they design an experiment?[55] In other words, they do not see a compound or element that makes GE plants different than the non-GE they could run a test on.

Nevertheless, there is a small amount of longitudinal and multigenerational feeding studies in animals in which scientists haven't observed any harm to animals caused by GE foods, and they use these results to suggest and justify that follow-up testing of GE crops in humans is unnecessary.

However, on closer look, you can see that not all these studies followed international standards, and they only lasted between 96 days and 104 weeks. Consequently, this raises a couple of important questions: when is the evidence sufficient enough to be conclusive? How long does a study have to be, or how many generations need to be examined to conclude that humans are not affected by GE?

More importantly is how GE may be altering the nonvisible aspects of the plant, like its life essence. Scientists are observing that the chemical compounds of GE plants are similar to non-GE, but they can't see if their life essence (energy) is the same. According to TCM, the genetic aspects of an organism functions within its life essence. Consequently, a change in its genetic composition (GE) may cause damage to its life essence. Therefore, damage to the life essence of our food produced by GE may not create damage to its nutrients. Instead it could cause dysfunction in its realm of influence (energetics) in humans, such as our vitality, fertility, immunity, hormonal function, higher awareness, and graceful aging.[54]

ALL FOODS ARE SUPERFOODS

As shocking as this may sound, there is no such thing as a superfood food group. Superfood is a marketing and media term assigned to food thought to be nutritionally dense and consequently good for your health. Some examples of foods labeled as superfoods are blueberries, goji berries, chia seeds, salmon, kale, and acai. However, there are no set criteria to determine what should be considered a superfood, and science does not recognize the term either. There are no regulations. Therefore, anyone can label a food *superfood* and market it as such.

It is a good idea to incorporate nutrient-dense foods such as these in your diet. Nonetheless, just because a food is labeled healthy or as a superfood, it does not mean you can eat—or even worse, supplement—unlimited quantities of it. Overeating (getting more than your body needs) superfoods or any other food will not give your body superpowers. It's quite the opposite. It can cause health issues such as weight gain, blood sugar imbalances, or health problems due to overconsumption of calories and one or more nutrients.

Excluding foods from our diet that are not labeled as superfoods is also a mistake because no one food contains a perfect balance of nutrients to sustain a healthy life. All foods labeled superfoods or not have a variety of nutrients and other health benefits that we need for the proper functioning of our bodies. Even iceberg lettuce, which is often regarded as not having any nutrients, has health benefits that include lower cholesterol levels, cancer prevention, neuroprotector, improved sleep, managed anxiety, lowered inflammation, and a constant supply of antioxidants.

Therefore, to be healthy, you should listen to your body and consume a variety of nutritious foods that are right for your current condition and in the right quantities. The model diet is one that is mostly plant-based with a wide range of fruits, vegetables, nuts, whole grains, and organic or free-range animal products (or any healthy vegetarian protein if you are vegan). Eating a balanced diet is key to good health, and no amount of superfood will save you or override your bad habits.

A balanced diet is one that gives your body the nutrients it needs to function correctly. For this reason, as much as possible, try to eat foods that are in season and local to your area. Seasonal foods bring us the nutrition that we need at that particular time of the year. For instance, spring is often wet and sticky in some parts of the world, which means we need food that can take away the dampness in our body, such as corn, white beans, and onion.

Summer is hot, so we need to eat food to cool us down, such as watermelon and cucumber. Autumn is dry, which means we need foods that moisturize and "lubricate," such as snow peas, pumpkin, and honey. Winter is cold, so we need food which warms up the body, such as soups, or beef.

Eating in-season food also means avoiding artificial ripening with gases or eating a bland version of a fruit or vegetable that has been shipped thousands of miles. Eating seasonally also results in the most nutrient-dense produce. Studies have shown that fruits and vegetables contain more nutrients when allowed to ripen naturally on their parent plant. Moreover, when we are in balance and feeling vital, eating what grows seasonally and regionally helps us maintain that balance.

Further, a balanced diet limits the consumption of empty calories, in other words, foods that provide little or no nutritional value, such as calories that come from sugars, refined products, and saturated fats, like butter and shortening.

The following nutrition pyramid (figure 2) serves as a guide for disease prevention and optimal health. It is a map that points in the direction toward habitual proper nutrition.

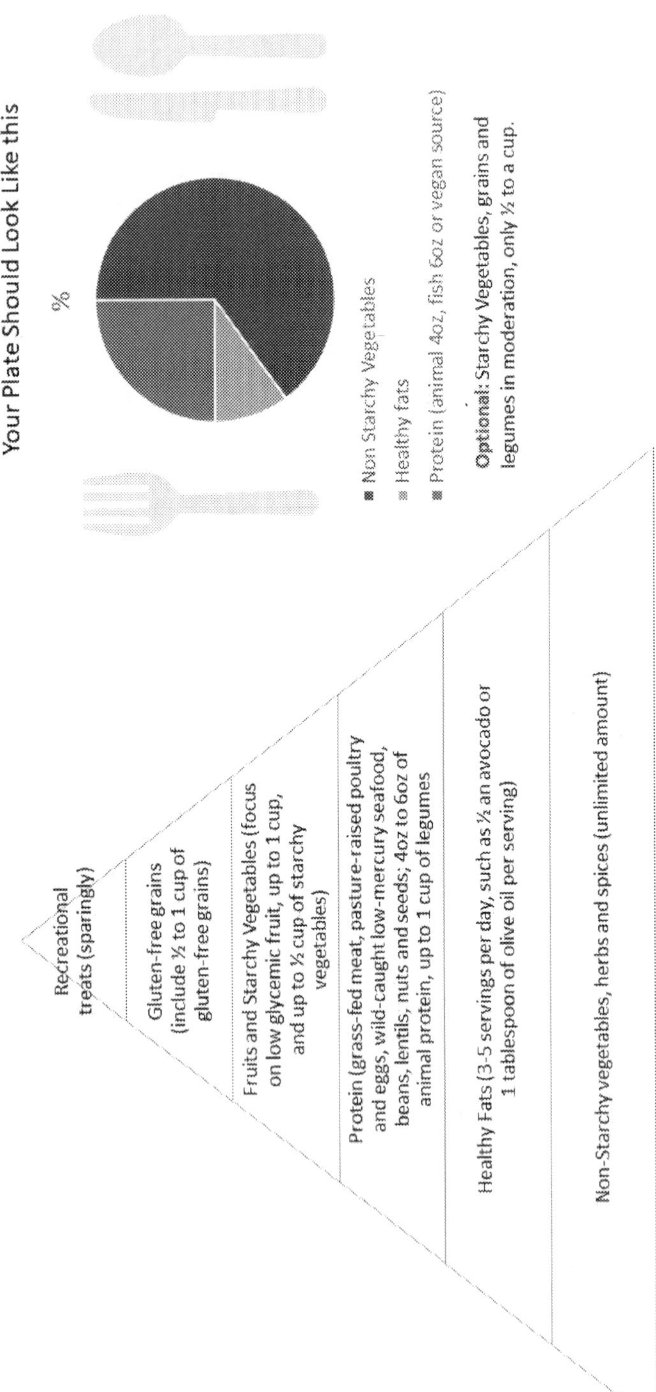

Figure. 2—Nutritional Pyramid.[54]

These percentages are appropriate for most people. However, depending on your current health condition, you may need to make adjustments. For example, if you are gluten-intolerant, you would not be able to eat gluten at this time. Instead eat non-glutenous grains. If you are very deficient and weak, then I recommend instead to work directly with me or another traditional medicine professional that can be your personal counselor and design a dietary protocol just for your needs. Nonetheless, the right food plan for you will still feature whole "living" foods that support your body while placing you in harmony with the world around you.

It is worth noting that, while food is one of the most important influences to health, it is not enough when applied in the lives of people who need emotional and spiritual transformation for self-love and clarity of mind. Awareness practices that help a person gain an emotional harmony that supports discipline, commitment, and the intention necessary for a long, joyful, and successful life are essential for a complete healing plan[54]. Such is the case of my friend Barbara, who healed herself from Crohn's disease using a whole food nutritional program and other traditional medicine techniques. This is her story.

> After graduating from college in 1985, I was diagnosed with Crohn's Disease, an autoimmune illness of the intestinal tract. Doctors prescribed medications to try to keep the symptoms under control, but I continued on a downward spiral of getting sicker and weaker. A few years later, a new treatment of using immunosuppressive medication was offered, but thankfully I had an epiphany of thought. I stopped believing Crohn's was incurable and that many things caused me to get sick like pieces in a puzzle, such as stress, improper diet, and having chicken pox at age 16. So, the same had to be true, there must be pieces for a puzzle that could make me well. All I had to do was find them.
>
> As soon as I arrived to this awareness, my first piece immediately came to me when someone handed me a book written by Dr. Robert Atkins on how to heal chronic diseases naturally, mainly via diet. I then went to his Complimentary Medicine Center in NYC. He got me off the medications and taught me how to eat healthier and to stop eating the foods causing the inflammation in

my gut. Eventually, I filled in the mental, emotional and spiritual pieces that were missing and have remained off medications for over 15 years now!

At age 55 I'm in the best shape of my life enjoying radiant health, happiness, and joy. I believe everyone can find their way back to health just like I did by discovering & putting together the pieces of their puzzle.

You can read more about Barbara's journey and tips for regaining your health, happiness & joy in her book *Solving The Crohn's & Colitis Puzzle: Piecing Together Your Optimal Picture of Optimal Health & Vitality.*

ALKALINE-FORMING FOODS

Your body is designed to work within a narrow pH range. According to a 2012 study published in the *Journal of Environmental Health*, balancing your body's pH through an alkaline diet can be beneficial in reducing morbidity and mortality from chronic diseases such as hypertension, diabetes, arthritis, vitamin D deficiency, and low bone density, amongst others.

Most of the food we eat has the potential to alter our pH. Our body's acid-base (pH) should be between 6.5 (slightly acidic) and 7.5 (slightly alkaline). Overacidity in the body occurs from consuming too many acid-forming foods and not enough alkalizing foods. While our bodies can easily handle an occasional acid load, long-term acid buildup can exhaust our available alkalizing reserves. Moreover, our bodies should be slightly alkaline to build an alkaline reserve for acid-forming conditions such as stress, lack of exercise, or poor diet.

It is important to note that not all acid-forming foods are bad. In fact, consuming healthy acid-forming foods is necessary for optimum health. It's merely a matter of balance. Acid-forming foods include most high-protein foods, such as meat, fish, eggs, and most legumes (beans and peas, except lentils, which are alkaline-forming). Sugar, coffee, alcohol, and most grains are also acid-forming. Alkaline-forming foods include nearly all vegetables and fruits, especially citrus, many nuts and seeds, spices, apple cider vinegar (with the mother), sprouts, cereal grasses, and herbs.

You can transform mildly acid-forming foods like whole grains and legumes by soaking them before cooking them. Soaking starts the sprouting process, which is alkalizing. Another way is to chew your food thoroughly, which is also highly alkalizing. It mixes your food with saliva, which is a very alkaline fluid. Additionally the chewing process serves as the first step to proper digestion and allows you to absorb more nutrients from food, helps you maintain a healthy weight, allows for easier absorption, and leads to fewer digestive issues like gas and bloating.

According to Dr. T. Katase, there is a relationship between the acid-alkaline balance and vitamins. Her studies showed the following associations:

- Vitamin B is useful in maintaining the alkaline-acid balance in the case of overeating protein. Foods that contain vitamin B include brown rice, barley, mochi (sweet rice), wheat, walnuts, sesame seeds, azuki beans (red beans), cabbage, burdock, green tea, and so on.

- Vitamin A occurs in the case of overeating fat. This vitamin can be found in liver, egg yolk, squash, shiso, celery, radish leaves, red pepper leaves, carrot, carrot leaves, scallion, parsley, green pepper, mugwort, nori, hijiki, wakame (sea vegetables), and so forth.

- Vitamin C occurs in the case of overeating carbohydrates and sugar. You can find this vitamin in citrus foods, red pepper, carrot leaves, parsley, spinach, persimmon leaves, green tea, and so on.

- Vitamin D relates to all of them. You can find vitamin D in large amounts in the following foods: all mushrooms in general, in particular, shiitake, yeast, cod liver oil, and any fish liver oil.

Note that, if you take too many vitamins in pill form, they can cause acidosis. On the other hand, vitamins from natural foods do not usually cause acidosis.[56] If you have the need to take supplements, buy those that are made by whole foods, such as the following brands: Health Force

Nutritionals, New Chapter, Nature's Plus, Garden of Life, and Natural Vitality, to name a few (in no particular order).

TWO FORGOTTEN FOODS: WHOLE WHEAT AND BROWN RICE

Both wheat and rice have gotten a bad rap in the last decade from the diet and health industry. We hear things like:

- I'm gluten intolerant.
- Carbs are bad for you.
- Blood sugar spikes when you eat carbs.
- If you want to lose weight, you can't eat carbs.
- Our ancestors did not eat grains.

And so on and so on. Although there is some truth to these statements, they are not entirely correct, and they are contributing to the malnourishment and health problems of this country.

Whole wheat is a remarkable food used in the traditional medicines of China and India to strengthen the body and nurture the mind and the heart. Unfortunately, in our Western culture, the form of wheat that we mostly consume is genetically modified, has been refined and stripped of its nutritional value, and has herbicide residue, leading to a society of autoimmune disorders and gluten intolerance.[53]

However, virtually no one is allergic to wheat in its whole form—before it's been milled into flour, also known as *wheat berries*. These berries, if grown in fertile soil (organic), are loaded with dozens of minerals and micronutrients. Two of the essential minerals that are stripped of wheat when it is refined are:

> Whole wheat is one of the best food sources of *selenium*. A few of the health benefits of selenium are:[54]

- Cancer prevention studies have demonstrated that cancer rates are lower in areas where selenium is abundant in the soil.
- Cancer studies also have shown that this mineral cuts cancer death rates by 50 percent!
- It keeps the thyroid healthy. Deficiency of this mineral causes hypothyroidism.
- It prevents obesity. A selenium deficiency slows down your metabolism
- Selenium counteracts the toxicity of heavy metals such as cadmium, inorganic mercury, methylmercury, thallium, and, to a limited extent, silver.
- Selenium deactivates (to make inactive) many viruses, including HIV.
- It prevents premature aging, heart disease, arthritis, and multiple sclerosis.

Approximately 70 percent of the United States population suffers from *magnesium* deficiency, yet you can find plenty of magnesium in foods such as legumes, vegetables (especially green vegetables), and most of whole grains and seeds. The health benefits of magnesium-rich foods are:

- It calms nerves and other emotional imbalances, such as irritability, depression, bipolar disorder, and PMS.
- It is a muscle relaxant.
- It soothes migraines, cramps, and spasms.
- It relieves constipation.
- It balances blood sugar in both diabetes and alcoholism.
- It strengthens the structure of the body and counteracts conditions such as chronic fatigue syndrome, fibromyalgia, arthritis, and osteoporosis.

- Magnesium helps control intracellular processes and maintains calcium equilibrium. Too much calcium without magnesium can lead to calcium to deposit in the soft tissue instead of the skeleton. This can lead to degeneration, in particular, in the kidneys, skeleton, heart, and vascular system (as it promotes coronary artery calcification). Excess calcium can also affect overall immunity and contributes to the development of Alzheimer's.

- Magnesium dilates coronary arteries and peripheral vessels, relaxes smooth muscle (like the heart), helps prevent blood clotting, and promotes a regular heartbeat.

Brown rice, like whole wheat, contains an abundance of nutrients, including magnesium, which is lost when is refined and made into white rice. (Asian countries partly mill their rice; consequently, it contains more nutrients than the white rice in the West.) Some of the health benefits of unrefined brown rice are:

- Brown rice balances blood sugar, and rice bran, the coating found on brown rice, has been found in studies to even lower blood sugar.

- Rice bran is one of the most nutrient-dense foods ever studied. It contains seventy antioxidants, including a unique form of vitamin E that is known to lower cholesterol.

- In studies, when fermented, rice bran has shown to increase the vitality and anti-stress effects of the internal organs, especially the adrenals, thymus, spleen, and thyroid.

- The polysaccharides in rice bran stimulate immunity, control blood sugar, and have been used in cancer therapy to destroy cancer cells and reduce tumors.

- The antioxidant gamma oryzanol is only found in substantial quantities in brown rice. It strengthens the muscles and converts fat into lean body mass.

- The glutathione peroxidase (GPx) enzyme found in brown rice reduces mucus excess, boosts respiratory function, and helps detoxify the body. It has also been used in the treatment of cirrhosis, rheumatoid arthritis, multiple sclerosis, acne, and asthma.

- Brown rice contains the enzyme superoxide dismutase, which has been used to treat cataracts, rheumatoid, and osteoarthritis.

- Coenzyme Q10, also found in brown rice, burns fat into energy; therefore, it reduces obesity. Coenzyme Q10 is commonly used in the treatment of angina, high blood pressure, and general heart disease. It also counteracts the side effects of type 2 diabetes by protecting the mitochondrial DNA. It has also been used to treat neurodegenerative issues such as Parkinson's, fibromyalgia, and Huntington's.

- The tannins (proanthocyanidins) in brown rice are one of the most potent antioxidants available; thus they protect against cancer and other degenerative disorders. Additionally they facilitate wound healing; strengthen the arteries, veins, and capillaries; and improve circulation.

- Brown rice contains lecithin, a substance essential for proper function of the brain. It has been used extensively to enhance brain activity and to improve attention and learning in children. It also has a calming effect; therefore, it reduces hyperactivity. Lecithin protects against the formation of gallstones, high blood pressure, and excess cholesterol.

- The supplement inositol hexaphosphate (IP_6) is extracted from brown rice, and it is currently used in cancer therapy. It is believed that it can be used in the treatment of cardiovascular disease, kidney stones, and immune disorders like AIDS. This nutrient can also be found in other grains, legumes, and most seeds.

Also in Eastern medicine, due to its high nutritional content, brown rice has a long history of being used for food therapy, in particular in the form of congee. Congee is a thin rice porridge consisting of a handful of rice simmered in five or six times the amount of water. Easy to digest, it is full of nutrients. Even though it can be used on its own, it can also be customized to help restore health according to each person's constitutional needs.

Rice is the traditional grain used for congees, but you can substitute with millet, spelt, or other nutritious grains. You can also add herbs such as ginger or astragalus to increase its potency. Congee has been used preventatively to promote good health and digestion for centuries. However, it is particularly helpful for those recovering from chemotherapy, any major illness, stomach and digestive disorders, or surgical procedures.

SIMPLE CONGEE RECIPE

Cook one cup of brown rice in six cups of water in a covered pot four to six hours on warm or use the lowest flame possible. A crockpot works great to make congee. It is better to use too much water than too little, and it is said that the longer it cooks the more powerful it is.

Note that minerals work best in relationship with all the other minerals found in whole, unrefined foods, as in the case of brown rice and whole wheat. Single minerals do not work well in isolation. For example, overconsumption of lecithin in isolation (as a supplement) can have serious side effects such as severe abdominal pain and weight loss.

SOAK YOUR GRAINS, NUTS, AND LEGUMES

The process of soaking grains and legumes, also known as culturing, is centuries old. The purpose of soaking is to help break down antinutrients, such as phytic acid, tannins, enzyme inhibitors, and hard-to-digest components of the grains, legumes, and nuts. And at the same time, it helps to release beneficial nutrients like vitamin B and minerals. Soaking also starts the sprouting process, which makes your food more alkalizing and easier to digest.

Phytic acid or IP_6 is a compound found in grains and legumes and has received a lot of unfavorable publicity lately. It is being vilified as a mineral absorption inhibitor. However, this supplement is frequently extracted from brown rice and used successfully in cancer therapy to inhibit tumor growth and cause cancer cells to go back to normal. IP_6 may also have applications in the treatment of cardiovascular disease, kidney stones, and immune system disorders. Nevertheless, you can neutralize IP_6 in grains in legumes by soaking them and discarding the soak water, sprouting, fermenting, and roasting.[54]

HOW LONG SHOULD YOU SOAK GRAINS, LEGUMES, AND NUTS?

As little as seven hours of soaking in warm water will neutralize a significant portion of phytic acid in grains and legumes and will vastly improve their nutritional benefits. Placing soaked kombu or kelp seaweed at the bottom of the pot when soaking increases the effectiveness of the process. Add one part seaweed for six or more parts grains or legumes.

Soaking is not as laborious or time-consuming as you may think it may be. It is effortless to do. All it takes is a little planning ahead, and I set my grains, legumes, and nuts to soak right before going to bed and rinse them in the morning when I wake up, making them ready for whenever I need to cook. The result is a highly nutritious and easy-to-digest whole-grain food with excellent flavor.

FOOD AND OUR EMOTIONS

Foods do not only affect our body. Our emotional health is strongly related to our brain health and chemistry. To function correctly, our brain requires a healthy supply of vitamins and nutrients. Additionally these nutrients are needed for healthy productions of hormones, cellular energy, neurotransmitters, antioxidants, DNA, and digestive substances.

Neurotransmitters such as serotonin and dopamine, which regulate mood, are made from amino acids. These chemical pathways also require vitamins and minerals as co-factors for their normal function. Nearly every vitamin and mineral deficiency can cause psychiatric symptoms such as depression, anxiety, irritability, and low-stress tolerance.

Candice B. Pert, PhD, states in her book *Molecules of Emotions* that happiness is what we feel when our biochemicals of emotions, the neuropeptides, and their receptors are open and flowing freely throughout the psychosomatic network, integrating and coordinating our systems, organs, and cells in a smooth and rhythmic movement. Physiology and emotions are inseparable. The foods we eat, the addictive substances we take, and the lifestyle we lead all affect the condition of the cells.[2]

In fact, "Every change in the physiological state is accompanied by an appropriate change in the mental emotional state, conscious or unconscious, and conversely, every change in the mental emotional state, conscious or unconscious, is accompanied by an appropriate change in the physiological state," states Elmer Green, Mayo Clinic physician.

Moreover, a healthy cell is permeable. This means that nutrients can be efficiently absorbed into the cell, and likewise the toxic by-products of metabolism can exit the cell efficiently. When the cell is in a healthy condition, the polarity of the cell is precise, meaning there is the right amount of intracellular potassium and magnesium and extracellular sodium and calcium. When the cell is healthy, a person functions optimally, both physically and emotionally. When the cell is open and permeable, you feel happy, energetic, and optimistic.

Candice Pert, PhD, says, "Happiness is our natural state; bliss is hardwired. Only when our systems get blocked, shut down, and disarrayed do we experience the mood disorders that add up to unhappiness in extreme."

On the other hand, when a cell is not healthy, it is not permeable. Therefore, the nutrients are less able to get into the cell, and toxic waste tends to build up inside. When a cell is closed off and blocked, a person can feel depressed, lacking in energy, and pessimistic. For that reason, the condition of the cells not only affect you physically but also emotionally.

HOW DO THE FOODS WE EAT AFFECT OUR MOODS?

Foods either promote the opening and expansion of a cell or block and contract. The foods that favor cell expansion are potassium-rich and high in water such as apples, pears, bananas, kiwis, peaches, plums, grapes, apricots, and dried fruits, along with green leafy vegetables, potatoes, parsley, celery, carrots, lettuce, peppers, cucumbers, squash, sweet potatoes, pumpkin, broccoli, cabbage, cauliflower, peas, and beans.

For the potassium to get inside a cell, it is necessary that is coupled with magnesium as magnesium and potassium travel best together, and magnesium keeps the potassium inside the cell. Magnesium is an essential mineral for mental health. In fact, the National Institute of Health (NIH) reports that one sign of magnesium deficiency is depression. Foods that are high in water also encourage the opening of the cells, as water is the delivery system that gets the nutrients to the cell and removes toxicity.

Good-quality protein also causes healthy oxidation as protein provides energy to the body. The importance of quality cannot be overemphasized. The highest quality food sources are those grown via the most natural methods and in the healthiest soil. Healthy soil contains a balance of many minerals and microorganisms and produces superior plants. *Wild* or *wildcrafted*, *biodynamic*, and *organic* are terms associated with foods grown with natural methods and in healthy soils.

Additionally, foods rich in *omega*-3 fats play a crucial role in the growth and proper functioning of our body. According to a study presented at the annual meeting of the American Psychosomatic Society, intake of omega-3 fatty acids is correlated with better mood and a positive outlook and contributes to improving the structure of the areas of the brain associated with emotions.

Foods that lead to the contraction and blocking of the cell are those high in sodium and calcium; refined sugars; dairy foods like milk, yogurt, ice cream, and cheese; and alcohol. For example, too much alcohol consumption encourages oxidation. The cells become more rigid and closed off, so the more one drinks alcohol, the more one needs to drink it. The closed-off cell is in a state of slow oxidation, which means the energy of the cell is depleted. Consequently it affects us on all levels—physical, mental, and emotional.

Similarly, an excess of the foods mentioned above also promote mental and physical inflammation and sometimes aggression. In some cases, substantial positive results in health and mood have been experienced just by eliminating processed sugars, other refined foods, and foods that contain chemical ingredients and preservatives.

AN EASTERN PERSPECTIVE ON NUTRITION—TELL ME WHAT YOU EAT, AND I WILL TELL YOU WHO YOU ARE

Whereas our Western view of food is based on chemistry, the Eastern view resembles alchemy and is not so much concerned with ingredients but instead with the underlying energetic properties that are released in our body through digestion. In Eastern medicine, it is said that all things are formed from *qi* (pronounced chee and sometimes spelled chi) and everything is determined or characterized by its qi, its vital force or energy.

Qi is a key concept in Chinese and Japanese medicine, and it is similar to the term *prana* (life force) of India and is known as *ki* in Japan. Qi is a vital essence found in all things, and it comprises the material and nonmaterial. I will refer primarily to its expression as energy, keeping in mind that energy and matter are changeable into one another.

In its pure form, qi is subtle and refined. It is a substance with no form (energy). On the other hand, matter is a condensed, slowed-down form of qi. The sources of qi in the body are from the food we eat, the air we breathe, and the essences of the kidneys, which some part of this qi we are born with.

How well we use qi from these sources will depend on our lifestyle and attitudes. Whatever manifests in our bodies will be an expression of how well we use qi. For example, a person that is graceful has harmonious qi. Weak people lack qi, strong people have abundant qi, and people with clear minds have refined, as opposed to confused, qi. The human body depends on qi, blood, and other essential substances that change, flow, and circulate in channels within the body, named meridians, and have no material form.

Qi that stagnates causes accumulations resulting in obesity, tumors, cysts, cancers, and viral and yeast-related diseases that usually arise with a sedentary lifestyle as well as refined and rich diets. Exercise, herbal therapy, yoga, qi gong, acupuncture, and awareness practices such as meditation are ways that we can clear obstructions and maximize qi.

Another way we can clear obstructions and maximize qi is through the food we eat. The subtle essences of food have movements and actions that follow the same pathways of qi (chi) in the body after food had been consumed. Likewise, in this theory, the nutritional value of food is stated as a set of energetic properties that describe the actions that food has on our body. Food is described as possessing qualities such as warming or cooling, flavors such as pungent or sweet, or as acting on our body in a specific way. An energetic viewpoint suggests that we not only absorb nutrients from food, but we also absorb their qualities such as texture, temperature, taste, smell, look, movement, and feelings of the food sources that we consume.[57]

HARMONIZING THE FIVE ELEMENTS WITH FOOD

The qualities of each of the foods we consume can be classified under each of the five elements. Therefore, we can use the five element system covered in chapter one to select specific foods that bring the energy of a particular element into our body to help harmonize our health and emotions. Each element has a corresponding emotional predisposition. The core emotional energies include the emotion of healthily balanced synergy and the emotional response to stress. (See details in chapter 1.)

According to this theory, there are seven human emotions: joy, anger, anxiety, melancholy, sorrow, fear, and fright. These emotions are human being's response to the external environment. In small amounts, they do not cause any physical ailments, but in large quantity and over prolonged periods, they can affect the proper functions of a person's internal organs.

It is important to recognize that emotional states arise in response to circumstances and perceptions. They are not inherently right or wrong. Our tendency to judge some feelings as good and others as bad is one of the leading impediments to freely experiencing and expressing emotions.

"If we could just feel what we feel and allow the natural transformation of emotional states, then we would find ourselves continuously re-entering the synergic or peaceful, harmonious state," writes Marsaa Teeguarden, psychotherapist and founder of Jin Shin Do.® "Acceptance is a key to entering or experiencing the synergic states."

On the other hand, researchers warn that emotional suppression can lead to potentially severe mental and physical health problems and even premature death.[58]

According to the ancient Chinese and Japanese, one human emotion can be curbed using another emotion based on the controlling cycle of the five elements (covered in chapter 1). For example, joy (fire) can overcome anxiety/sorrow (metal), which in turn can overcome anger (wood). Anger (wood) can overcome melancholy (earth), which in turn can overcome fear (water). Each element is associated with a pair of organs and different kinds of emotions. We can look to see if a deficiency or excess of one of the elements could be contributing to physical health or emotional issue and then attempt to resolve this by adjusting our diet. (For an explanation of the five element cycle, review chapter 1.)

To balance emotions with food, we need to consider foods regarding which of the five element energy they might increase inside our body. As previously noted in chapter 1, a detailed look at five element theory is beyond the scope of this book. Nevertheless, to give you an idea of how to use this system to harmonize your emotions, below is a basic summary and only contains a few examples of foods and feelings associated with each element.

THE WOOD (AIR) ELEMENT

Energy pathways: Liver and gallbladder

Emotional energy: Assertion. The liver is often likened to making long-term plans and strategies. At the same time, the liver is responsible for establishing a smooth flow in the body and emotions.

Balanced: When the liver is harmonious, a person tends to be calm with clear judgment and capable of decisive action. It also includes self-assertion, motivation, the will to become, creativity, response-ability, the ability to respond appropriately, and kindness.

Wood/air disharmony: A classic indication of liver disharmony is emotional difficulty related to anger. Typically mood swings, as well as emotional excesses, may be associated with liver disharmony. Anger and frustration may change into a range of distressed emotional states, from the excess manifestations of irritability, impatience, resentment, animosity, belligerence, indignation, bitterness, and vengefulness, to the expressions of guilt, self-blame, lack of motivation, apathy, boredom, impotence, and depression. Starting many projects or tasks without completing them is also often associated with a liver disharmony.

Harmonizing foods: Barley, wheat, rye, rising greens (leeks, onions, celery, sprouts), spring fruits

THE FIRE ELEMENT

Energy pathways: Heart, pericardium, small intestine, and triple warmer

Emotional energy: Joy. Not to confuse joy with happiness, you can think of it more as enthusiasm for living. It is the abundant overspilling spirit of the heart, reaching out to life. Laughter is the sound of the fire element, and laughter generally is beneficial to the heart.

Balanced: When fire is in harmoniums, a person experiences happiness, self-confidence, and compassion.

Fire disharmony: The extreme emotions of fire are overjoy or overexcitation and shock/fright. These are stressors to the heart. Change is stressful. Whether it is a negative stress such as the heartbreaking end of a love relationship or a positive stress such as winning the big lottery, events, situations, and feelings, which require a significant readjustment to take place, exert stress and strain on the heart. The heart is vulnerable to emotional extremes. In excess or hyperactivity, the distressed emotional states of fire include hypertension, elation, restlessness, nervousness, anxiety, and hysteria. Deficient distress states include sadness, discouragement, self-doubt, despair, emptiness, hopelessness, and depression. Inappropriate laughter or the complete absence of laughter may signal fire imbalance.

Harmonizing foods: Corn, amaranth, quinoa, large, leafy greens (kale, collards, dandelion), summer fruits

THE EARTH ELEMENT

Energy pathways: Spleen, pancreas, stomach

Emotional energy: The balanced or synergic emotion of the earth element is sympathy and empathy.

Balanced: Earth harmonious states are consideration and recollection. This is the energy of stepping outside of self-interest with genuine concern for others. This emotional-spiritual inclination of earth is concerned with deep, feeling connection.

Earth disharmony: Worry or overconcern, pity or over sympathy, and pensiveness or excessive thinking and reminiscence are the extreme emotions of the earth phase. The spectrum of hyperactive distress includes overthinking, worry, brooding, selfishness, self-absorption, anxiety, and obsessiveness. Mental fatigue, poor concentration, forgetfulness, indifference, blaming, victim mentality, and alienation are some of the distressed responses in the deficient earth energy.

Harmonizing foods: Millet, round vegetables (squash, pumpkin, cabbage, cauliflower), late summer fruits

THE METAL ELEMENT (ETHER)

Energy pathways: Lungs, large intestine

Emotional energy: The metal element is concerned with allowing/receiving and releasing.

Balanced: When metal is harmonious, a person is concerned with openness, receptivity, independence, and nonattachment.

Metal disharmony: The extreme emotions of metal are grief, sorrow, and lamentation. These are painful emotions arising from loss. The all-too-common dysfunctional response, leading to distressed states, is to cling to the suffering, to hold on tightly and not let go of the past, or to shut down and not feel at all. The distressed states of metal are excessive grieving, stoicism, defensive pride, possessiveness, jealousy, envy, and greed. The deficient spectrum includes self-pity, hypersensitivity, denial, withholding of emotion, deprivation, despondency, and oppression.

Harmonizing foods: Rice, contracted plants, roots (radish, onion, burdock, carrot), autumn fruits

THE WATER ELEMENT

Energy pathways: Kidneys, urinary bladder

Emotional energy: Water contains the life principle of flow, adaptability, and flexibility, but also the qualities of power and form.

Balanced: When water is harmonious, a person can go with the flow, follow his or her dreams (purpose), and adapt to changing circumstances without any issues. They also are able to exert caution when is appropriate.

Water disharmony: Unreasonable fear is often listed as the emotional aspect of water. The synergic feelings of the water phase are apprehension, resolution, volition, and trust. In distress states, the excess spectrum includes bravado, audacity, foolhardiness, superiority, suspicion, mistrust, and paranoia. The range of deficiency manifestations includes inadequacy, timidity, inferiority, fearfulness, panic, and phobias.

Harmonizing foods: Buckwheat, beans, seaweeds (cooked), winter and dried fruits

According to this theory, you can bring balance and health to your body by balancing these elements following the five element generating sequence or cycle described in chapter 1. For example:

- To increase the presence of wood energy, we might eat more steamed green vegetables.
- To experience more fire energy, we could eat more fire foods and include onions, garlic, and ginger in the dish.

- To feel more earth energy, we can experiment with more pumpkin and carrot soups and stewed apples for dessert.
- To increase the presence of metal energy, we might try more pressure-cooked brown rice, barley, and wheat.
- To experience more water energy, we can eat miso soups and bean and vegetable stews.

Similarly, we could reduce our exposure to specific element energy by eating less of the element foods associated with that element. So, if we felt too withdrawn, less metal energy foods and more fire energy foods could help.

This is a concept that most Westerners, including my clients, have a difficulty understanding. The question that often arises is why I am asking them to avoid or minimize certain foods that are healthy from a Western perspective. This happens because they are only looking at food for their nutritional value—the vitamins, minerals, fats, proteins, carbohydrates, antioxidants, and so forth—rather than observing the health benefits of food characterized by their energetic effects on the body and mind.

The benefit to understanding food energetics is to develop a more holistic perspective on nutrition. When it comes to our health, there is a risk in focusing only on the nutritional value of food and overlooking the energetic properties. For example, in the West, fruits are thought to be healthy because they have many great nutritional qualities, such as antioxidants that help fight cancer. They also improve mood and energy and support overall health and wellness. However, in Eastern medicine, overeating sweet, cold, raw foods like fruits are known to create dampness, which isn't a problem when eaten in moderation.

With this in mind, overeating fruits cause dampness in the body, including in the intestines, and dampness in the intestines eventually causes chronic diseases to form like candida, a fungal infection that thrives in damp environments and can be difficult to eliminate. Also candida causes many bothersome symptoms from rashes to brain fog, chronic fatigue, allergies to food, lethargy, and more.

As you can see, if we only consider the Western nutritional value of food such as fruits, eating a lot of fruits seems to be a good thing to do for our health. However, when taking into consideration the energetic perspective of fruit, it becomes apparent that, if we want to stay healthy, we should only eat fruit in moderation.

It is important to note that these two worldviews are not at odds with each other. Instead they complement each other, and together they can help us understand a fundamental principle in creating radiant, lifelong health, which is balance and moderation.

THE FOUNDATION OF GOOD NUTRITION: BALANCE AND MINDFULNESS

Healthy nutrition doesn't need to be about rigorous control. A constant obsession with optimal eating creates distress and anxiety around strict nutrition goals, and those persistent negative emotions may lead to health issues. It is impossible for any of us to eat the perfect diet all the time. Instead, do the best you can, and as much as possible, let your thoughts about food be positive ones. Let food be a source of pleasure, nourishment, and nutrients rather than stress and confusion.

It is essential to read labels, understand where your food comes from, and pay attention to how the food you eat affects your body. But it's equally important to be aware of trying to eat perfectly is causing you so much stress that it might have a negative impact on your health.

Rather than obsessing on what you are eating, when making food choices, it is healthier to pay attention and be fully conscious of what is happening both inside and outside yourself—in your body, heart, and mind—and your surroundings. Do not compare yourself to anyone else. And do not judge yourself or others. Just witness the many sensations and thoughts that come up and make an informed aware decision of what is the best choice of food for you at that moment.

Ideally, find healthy and nourishing foods that are also satisfying and comforting. However, do not stress about it. As you practice eating healthier and a variety of food, you will be less inclined to binge on unhealthy comfort foods and more willing to enjoy healthy foods, ultimately finding many foods mentally and physically satisfying as opposed to just a few.

More importantly, balance of mind and serenity are essential when making food choices and sustaining health. Slowing down is one of the best ways we can get our mind and body to communicate what we need for nutrition. Simple ways to slow down might include sitting down to eat, chewing each bite twenty-five times (or more), and setting your fork down between bites.

In particular, multitasking while eating does not allow you to listen deeply to your body's needs and wants. When we are distracted, it is harder to listen to our body's signals about food and emotional needs. As much as possible, try eating with no TV, phones, or other distractions other than enjoying the conversation with whom you are sharing your meal.

Finally practice an attitude of gratitude. Pause for a minute or two before you begin eating to contemplate everything and everyone it took to bring the meal to your table. Also silently express your gratitude for the opportunity to enjoy this delicious food and the time you get to spend with the people you are sharing a meal.

At the end of the day, you are the only real expert on your body and your health. Doctors, holistic health practitioners, and nutritionists can share information, but only you know what foods are right for you.

For this reason alone, it is crucial for you to slow down and listen to your body.

CHAPTER FOUR

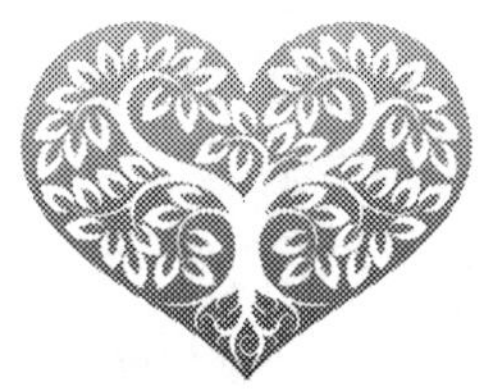

The Role of Herbs in Healing

All that man needs for health and healing has been provided by God in nature, the challenge of science is to find it.

—PHILIPPUS THEOPHRASTRUS BOMBAST THAT OF AUREOLUS-PARACELSUS (1493–1541)

In general, an herb is a plant or plant part used for its scent, flavor, or therapeutic properties. However, in ancient times, the category of herbs could include not only plants but also animals and minerals. In other words, the definition of an herb was any natural product that was ingested or applied externally to an individual to prevent and heal physical illnesses by balancing the flow of qi (vital energy) and supplying suitable materials for regeneration of body cells or tissues.

Herbs are foods with discrete, particular, and often strong qualities and disagreeable taste or smell that can aid significantly in every aspect of healing. Since herbs fall into the category of strong foods, just like regular foods, they are an extension of traditional medicine's second secret to health and longevity.

Considering regular food represents only a small part of our food dominion, a person can eat a healthy diet and still be lacking in some vitamins, minerals, amino acids, and other substances that nourish some parts of the body and regenerate specific tissues or cells. as a result, in traditional medicine, herbs are often used to supplement the diet and to prevent disease and support health.

Humans have been using herbs for healing for thousands of years. Ancient Taoist, Chinese, and Egyptian papyrus writings describe medicinal uses for plants as early as 3000 BC. Indigenous cultures, such as African and Native American, used herbs in their healing rituals, while others such as Ayurveda and TCM have developed complete traditional medical systems in which herbal therapies were used.

Herbal medicine aims to return the body to a state of natural balance so it can start healing itself. Plants have been humanity's primary medicine for centuries, and herbalism has been practiced to remedy or alleviate many conditions, such as allergies, asthma, eczema, PMS, migraines, menopausal symptoms, chronic fatigue, IBS, and cancer, among others. A significant benefit of herbal medicine is that it is safer and sometimes even more effective than synthetic pharmaceuticals. On the other hand, according to the *Journal of American Medical Association*, adverse reactions to medicines are the fourth-leading cause of death in the United States. Herbal supplements do work and are highly effective, but only if you are using high-quality ingredients that are given in the right quantity.

Moreover, plants possess attributes that pharmaceuticals never will. Their chemistry is highly complex, and instead of providing a single chemical to treat, herbs often contain hundreds to thousands of compounds working together synergistically. In fact, an active ingredient of a plant can become less safe or effective, if used in isolation from the rest of the plant. According to herbal medicine experts, the effect of the whole plant is more significant than its parts, and a entire herb may contain protective compounds or exert some positive side effects, which will improve other health problems that one does not expect it to address.

For example, although meadowsweet contains salicylic acid, it is used to treat stomach ulcers, which taken in isolation (like aspirin, which originated from this plant) can induce stomach ulcers. However, the whole meadowsweet herb naturally contains other compounds that counteract the irritant qualities of salicylic acid. The complex compounds within plants work in synergy with each other and, if used adequately, cause very few, if any, side effects of any sort.

In addition, herbs can act on the body as powerfully as synthetic drugs. Therefore, treat them with the same care and respect as you would any other medication. Not unlike synthetic drugs, herbs may cause allergic reactions or adverse effects specific to an individual if they are of poor quality, adulterated, or confused with other herbs that may be toxic when misused or alongside prescription medication without being checked for possible interactions.

In general, herbal supplements are very safe and effective. However, when taking medication, you should investigate possible interactions with an herbal remedy you may be considering consuming. Be careful about mixing herbs and drugs that have similar actions. Similarly, avoid combining herbs and drugs that have opposing effects.

Additional considerations when ingesting herbal supplements are:

- Herbs that can thin blood, such as dong quai, feverfew, garlic, and ginger, could cause problems if taken before surgery. It is best to stop taking any of these herbs at least ten to fourteen days before surgery.
- Herbs that have an effect on the nervous system like kava and valerian may increase the effects of anesthesia. Stop taking any of these herbs at least a week before surgery.
- Unless you're under the care of a knowledgeable practitioner, avoid taking any herbs during pregnancy, in particular during the first trimester. Exception: it's considered safe to take up to 1,000 milligrams of ginger in capsule or candied forms for morning sickness. Short-term use of echinacea seems safe for pregnant women who develop colds or flu.

- Breastfeeding women should avoid most medicinal herbs for the first four to six months of a baby's life. An exception is herbs that can stimulate breast milk production such as fenugreek, blessed thistle, vitex, and alfalfa.

- Herbal remedies that are safe for adults may not be safe for children; therefore, ask a knowledgeable practitioner for advice on herbs that are safe for children and the appropriate dose.

Typical herbal preparations are sold as tablets, capsules, powders, teas, salves, creams, liniments, syrups, extracts, and fresh or dried plants. All herbs may be purchased and consumed individually. However, it is more practical and effective to use a formula that was designed for you or your specific condition. That is why a personalized herbal supplement is a valuable service I provide to my clients.

HERBAL FORMULAS—THE SUM IS GREATER THAN ITS PARTS

As an herbalist, I generally favor formulas instead of simples (a single herb) because years of clinical experience have shown they offer more significant health benefits and optimal therapeutic efficacy. Formulas combine individual herbs that are designed to strengthen and balance one another's effects, providing a more holistic outcome. This means most herbs in a formula create a unique synergy. Therefore, the level of support offered by a formula is amplified since a formula is more effective than the sum of its parts.

Additionally the interactions between the components of different formulas are thought to produce specific synergistic effects on multiple organ systems, thus improving the pharmacological activities and reducing the adverse clinical reactions caused by some individual herbs. In formulas, each herb complements the others, and together they support your body in its path to health. Moreover, a significant advantage of formulas is that they can also be designed specifically for your unique needs, consequently making it more accurate for your constitution and condition.

Furthermore, except for in herbal shamanism, herbal formulas are more historically representative of herbal medicine. The present-day popular overuse of single herbs may be due to modern Western herbalism's correlating conventional medicine's symptomatic approach to healing. We are used to the philosophy of one pill for the one condition, that is, the use of aspirin/willow bark for pain, antibiotics/echinacea for infections, and stimulants/ginseng for fatigue.

Note that I'm not discounting the effectiveness of using single herbs. I've seen them work very well, especially for acute conditions and when carefully chosen by an experienced herbalist.

WHY I USE HERBAL TINCTURES/EXTRACTS OVER OTHER TYPES OF PREPARATIONS

Teas, capsules, pills, and extracts are all made from the same combination of herbs. However, the most effective herbal supplements are going to be the ones that a person can realistically take, and I will be honest that most therapeutic dosages of herbs do not taste like candy. Therefore, people have a hard time drinking large quantities of medicinal tea. Not to mention, in this busy world, people do not have the time to brew a batch of medicinal tea every day. Instead most people prefer quick and easy medication.

As for capsules and pills, unless they are concentrated, you will need to take a large quantity to get the same medicinal effects as one dose of an extract (about twelve pills two or three times per day). Additionally pills and capsules will have to be digested before they reach the bloodstream and take effect, and in some cases, the age and medical condition of a person may influence how much herb will make it to the bloodstream after digestion. More importantly, when taking capsules and pills, you need to consider if there are binders in them that may make them less absorbable or make them an allergen to you.

On the other hand, tinctures are concentrated, easy, and convenient to use, as nothing needs to be brewed. Because they are in liquid form, they enter the bloodstream much more directly and faster than by any other means. Therefore, the action in the body is usually faster. Although some herbs will have an immediate effect, such as those used to help you relax, others that are more nutritive and building in nature may take several weeks of continual use before best results are seen. Other advantages of herbal tinctures and extracts are:

- In general, one teaspoon of an herbal extract is equal to an eight-ounce cup of medicinal tea.
- Mostly, tinctures/extracts take effect within ten to fifteen minutes of taking them, whereas capsules will need to be digested before you start seeing the results.
- Only a small amount is needed to obtain medicinal effects.
- Extracts are easy to give to children since they must take only small amounts and most children do not enjoy drinking tea or can take capsules.
- It is easy to carry a bottle of tincture in your purse and have it available to you at all times.
- Even though people enjoy taking herbs in the form of syrups, they are often not as potent as tinctures.
- Tinctures also have a long shelf life (much longer than the dried herb alone would have) and are incredibly stable if stored correctly.

Please note that there are times where a medicinal tea will be more appropriate than a tincture. In particular, when a water-soluble constituent of an herb is needed, such as the case with broken bones where you will need the silica and other minerals of the plant, in the case of some digestive and lung disorders.

HOW TO MAKE HERBAL TINCTURES AT HOME

Tinctures are liquid extracts made from herbs. They are usually extracted in alcohol; although you can extract herbs using vinegar and glycerin as well. Making tinctures or herbal extracts is both an art and a science. It seems simple but is not, in particular, if using the weight-to-volume (scientific) method of extraction. However, when making tinctures at home, the easiest way to make a tincture is to use the folk method. This method requires no measuring, and it is suitable for general use (but not recommended for professional use).

Next, I will describe the folk method. It is an effective way of creating extracts without using the scientific method, which is more effective and accurate. The only supplies you will need are herbs, glass mason jars, cotton muslin bags, and a coffee grinder. You can use fresh or dried herbs

The percent of alcohol (alcohol-to-water ratio) to use will depend on the type of material you are working with. The standard for most tinctures is to use 40 to 50 percent alcohol (80- to 90-proof vodka). It can be used to extract both dried and fresh herbs. It works well with herbs that are not juicy and with water-soluble properties

To extract mucilage herbs, you will need to use 25 percent alcohol. Mucilaginous herbs have a slippery mild taste and swell in water, producing a gellike mass such as marshmallow, slippery elm, and mullein. The easiest way to calculate is to use 60 percent water of the total amount of liquid that you will need to make the tincture using 40 percent alcohol (vodka). For example, if you need ten ounces of fluid, use six ounces of water and four ounces of vodka.

67 to 70 percent is commonly used for herbs with volatile and aromatic properties and high-moisture herbs such as lemon balm, berries, and aromatic roots like cinnamon. The easiest way to calculate is to use half of the amount you need of 80-proof vodka and add half of 190-proof grain alcohol.

For resins such as myrrh and herbs that have essential oils that do not dissipate easily like rosemary, use 85 to 95 percent (190-proof grain alcohol). This is not the most common type of extraction.

Grind dried herbs using a coffee grinder or blender to release juice and expose surface area. If you are using a coffee grinder, use it exclusively to grind herbs. Otherwise all your extracts will smell like coffee. Fresh herbs should be chopped with a knife instead of using a coffee grinder.

Now fill jars with herbs. If you are using with leaves and flowers, if fresh, only fill up to two thirds to three fourths of the jar. If you are working with dried herbs, just fill the jar one half to three fourths with herb. If you are using with roots, barks, and berries, if fresh, just fill up to one third to one half of the jar. If you are working with dried herbs, just fill the jar one fourth to one thirds with herbs.

Next pour alcohol to the top of the jar to cover herbs completely. Close the jar and store in a dark, dry place. Shake the jar twice a day for at least two weeks and up to six to eight weeks.

Now is the time to press. Drape a muslin bag (or cheesecloth) over a strainer, and put the strainer on top of a glass container large enough to hold the amount of tincture being pressed. Allow to drip as much as you can. Then squeeze and twist the muslin bag until all the tincture has been extracted (or as much as you are able to get out). Finally pour the contents of tincture into an amber glass bottle. Label your container with the name of the herb and extraction date. Store your tincture in a cool, dark place. It will keep for many years.

Use only organic or wildcrafted herbs and from a reliable source like, Pacifical Botanicals, or Start-West botanicals (in no particular order)

REASONS WHY HERBS MAY NOT HAVE WORKED IN THE PAST FOR YOU

I can't emphasize enough: herbal supplements work and are highly effective if you use and prepare them correctly. And they are an excellent alternative to the toxic medications that exist today with none or very minimum side effects.

The following are the main reasons why people do not have success working with herbs:

- This sounds silly and illogical, but one of the main reasons that herbal supplements do not work has to do with people buying the products and not taking them on a consistent basis. Like any other medication, herbs need to be taken consistently to work. However, there are individuals not able to accommodate a change in their lives even if it means that taking an herbal supplement or changing their diet will help them heal.

- People are not taking the necessary amount for the herbal supplement to be medicinal, or it's an inaccurate preparation. The directions of most over-the-counter herbal supplements list a small dose that is rarely medicinal. The dose of herbs you take will vary depending on your goal and condition. Dosage also depends on if you have chronic or acute symptoms. A knowledgeable professional should be able to guide you on how much to take of an herbal supplement. However, below are some guidelines that you can follow:

    - Tinctures or extracts: Ingest usually thirty to sixty drops (the equivalent of one to two droppers full), two to five times a day, or one teaspoon two times a day (about two hundred drops). The amount will depend on the formula and your condition. In general, acute conditions require smaller dosages and to be taken more times per day than chronic conditions. However, if you are under the supervision of an experienced practitioner, you might be asked to take up to a tablespoon two or three times a day, especially for those in pain such as migraines or nerve/muscle pain.

        - Children's dosage guide by age (consult a professional before administering herbal supplements to children)

          Age two to three: ten drops
Age three to four: twelve drops
Age four to six: fifteen drops
Age six to nine: twenty drops
Age nine to twelve: twenty-four drops
Twelve and over: thirty to sixty drops

    - Teas: Mix a half-ounce (equivalent of seven regular size tea bags) of dried herb in two cups of water daily. Infused or decoct for at least twenty minutes. You will need to buy fifteen ounces of dried herb for a monthly supply.

    - Syrups: Give in one teaspoon to one tablespoon doses, two to three times a day.

  - o Capsule and pills: Follow the directions on the box.

- The third most important factor in taking herbs is how long they should be taken. If you have an acute health condition, like a cold, a bruise, or a simple rash, then you are going to take herbs for at least twenty-four to forty-eight hours before stopping. If you have a chronic long-term health problem, you are going to have to take the herbal supplements for many weeks or months or until your health has been restored. It takes years to develop a chronic condition. Therefore, even if you feel better, it might take years to recover fully. I have seen it with my clients. Treatment usually takes between three and six months. However, people with severe conditions may take between eighteen and twenty-four months to fully recover.

- The quality and effectiveness of organic herbs are higher than nonorganic herbs. Also, if you are using herbs that are made from herb medicines or are old or stored improperly, you might not be getting the same medicinal properties as those that are organic and fresh. Always buy organic and from a reliable company such as Herb-Pharm, Gaia Herbs, or my brand, Moongazing Herbal Apothecary. The quality of the herb is directly correlated to its effectiveness.

EXPLORE THE MEDICINAL MAGIC IN YOUR KITCHEN.

"Let thy food be thy medicine and thy medicine be thy food," said Hypocrites.

You do not have to be a master herbalist or learn how to create sophisticated herbal formulas to experience the benefits of herbs. A lot of what we call herbs are everyday foods and spices that we can find in our kitchen, and as such, you can incorporate them into your diet or make into teas for prevention and treatment of acute and chronic conditions. For example, chicken soup contains thyme, garlic, and cayenne.

All antimicrobial herbs and the spices in chai tea provide a rich source of antioxidants and nutrients that support digestion and immunity, balance blood sugar, and combat inflammation. It has also been suggested that some of the spices in chai tea have antibacterial and anticancer effects.

Unfortunately modern-day commercialized chai beverages tend to be sugar-laden and more of a health threat than a health benefit. When buying prepared chai tea, pay attention to the ingredients on the labels, or better yet, skip the coffee shop, and make your own from scratch like in this recipe.

HEALTHY CHAI TEA

This will make about five cups worth, and it's caffeine-free, so your kids can drink it too.

Bring four cups of water or milk substitute, such as almond or coconut milk to a boil. Then lower the heat to a gentle simmer and add all the ingredients listed below. Cover with a secure lid and continue gentle simmer for twenty minutes. Then turn off the heat and let it sit. You can drink it right away, but the longer it sits, the better it tastes.

INGREDIENTS

Spices: 10 whole cloves, 12 whole cardamom pods, 12 whole black peppercorns, 2 cinnamon sticks, and 4 slices fresh ginger root (chopped)

1 cup coconut milk, soy milk, rice milk, or almond milk

Raw honey, agave, or stevia to taste

If you want a caffeinated version of chai tea, add one organic unflavored black or green tea bag to each hot serving. Steep for five minutes. Discard tea bag before serving.

A spice rack can be a powerful healing tool. Culinary herbs and spices are some of the healthiest foods on the planet and have strong therapeutic effects. Using culinary herbs and spices for healing is nothing new. TCM and Indian Ayurvedic systems have recognized the healing benefits of spices for thousands of years and used them for the maintenance of health and in the prevention, improvement, or treatment of physical and mental illness.

Some health benefits are unique to each spice, and others are shared among different spices. In fact, a study published in the *Journal of Medicinal Foods* found a direct correlation between the antioxidant phenol content of many spices and their ability to prevent heart disease and premature aging. According to this study, the spices that have the most phenol are cloves, cinnamon, allspice, oregano, marjoram, sage, thyme, tarragon, and rosemary.

Spices also help us digest food, detoxify our bodies, and keep our hearts and minds active. Not only are they excellent in meals for added flavor, they also provide vitamins and minerals and are critical to the nutritional density in foods you eat. Because of their nutrient density, they are thermogenic, meaning they naturally increase metabolism. Therefore, you can easily boost the nutritional value of your meals by merely adding spices.

Most of you have a spice rack filled with seasonings you use every day for cooking, but what do you know about their medicinal properties? In case you are not familiar with them, the following is a list of the most common herbs and spices that are found in your kitchens and their medicinal effects.

Herb/Spice	Health Benefits
Basil	Basil is antibacterial, anti-inflammatory, and a good source of magnesium. It promotes cardiovascular health because of its high content of vitamin A through its concentration of carotenoids such as beta-carotene. It is called "pro-vitamin A." Basil oil applied to the skin helps prevent pimples and contains anti-aging properties. It is rich in antioxidants.

Cayenne	Cayenne is anti-irritant, anticancer, antimicrobial, antifungal, and anti-allergen. It prevents migraines. It is a digestive aid and useful for blood clots. It is used for detox support and relieves joint pain. It supports weight loss and promotes heart health. Studies at Loma Linda University found that cayenne pepper may help prevent lung cancer in smokers.
Cardamom	Cardamom is aphrodisiac, antispasmodic, anticancer, anti-asthmatic, and anti-inflammatory. It is used for detoxification and improves blood circulation. It provides nausea and vomiting relief. It provides gastrointestinal protection, controls cholesterol, offers relief from cardiovascular issues, and improves blood circulation.
Cinnamon	Cinnamon is antispasmodic, antiemetic, antidiarrheal, anti-inflammatory, and antifungal. It helps fight infections like the common cold, loss of appetite, and erectile dysfunction (ED). Cinnamon may lower blood sugar in people with type 1 or type 2 diabetes. It reduces LDL cholesterol. Buy Ceylon Cinnamon whenever possible. It comes from Sri Lanka and is widely considered to be the best in the world.
Clove	Clove is aphrodisiac, anti-inflammatory, antiseptic, and antifungal. It relieves respiratory infections, improves digestion, and provides pain relief. It is high in antioxidants and a good source of minerals, particularly manganese, omega-3 fatty acids, fiber, and vitamins.

Coriander Coriander is antifungal and antiseptic. It lowers cholesterol and acts as an anti-inflammatory for the skin. It is also a digestive aid and reduces blood pressure. Coriander or cilantro is also an excellent source of dietary fiber, manganese, and iron. Coriander leaves are rich in vitamin C, vitamin K, and protein. They also contain small amounts of calcium, phosphorous, potassium, thiamin, niacin, and carotene.

Dill Dill boosts digestive health and reduces insomnia, hiccups, diarrhea, dysentery, menstrual disorders, respiratory disorders, and cancer. It can protect from bone degradation and is anti-inflammatory. Dill has a significant amount of vitamin A and vitamin C as well as trace amounts of folate, iron, and manganese.

Fennel The iron, phosphorous, calcium, magnesium, manganese, zinc, and vitamin K content in fennel all contribute to building and maintaining bone structure and strength. Fennel speeds up metabolism, aids digestion, increases iron absorption, and is estrogenic (promotes estrogen production). It is an excellent source of vitamin C and is anti-inflammatory. Ground fennel starts to lose its flavor after six months, while whole fennel seeds keep for three years. So it's best to buy whole and grind as needed.

Garlic Garlic is antimicrobial, anti-inflammatory, and antifungal. Garlic reduces blood pressure, improves cholesterol levels, helps prevents Alzheimer's disease and dementia, may increase longevity, improves athletic performance, detoxifies heavy metals in the body, and may improve overall health. Garlic is low in calories and very rich in vitamin C, vitamin B_6, and manganese.

Ginger Ginger is anti-nausea, anti-inflammatory, and anticancer. It reduces morning sickness, decreases muscle pain and soreness, can help with osteoarthritis, lowers blood sugar, reduces heart disease risks, treats chronic indigestion, decreases menstrual pain, lowers cholesterol levels, protects against Alzheimer's disease, and helps fight infections.

Mint Mint reduces seasonal allergy symptoms and fights the common cold, indigestion, depression, fatigue, memory loss, and irritable bowel syndrome (IBS). It is a breath freshener as well as a antiseptic and anti-carcinogen. Mint relieves nausea, headache, respiratory disorders, cough, and asthma. It helps with weight loss and oral care and increases mother's milk.

Nutmeg Nutmeg provides pain relief, soothes indigestion, improves cognitive function, detoxifies the body, boosts skin health, alleviates oral conditions, helps with insomnia, increases immune system function, helps prevent leukemia, and improves blood circulation and brain health. It is an aphrodisiac.

Oregano Oregano provides immune support. It is antifungal, antibacterial, anti-inflammatory, and anti-cancer. It is useful for respiratory infections. Research has shown essential oils from oregano may kill the foodborne pathogen listeria and the superbug MRSA, making it a valuable addition to hand soaps and disinfectants.

Parsley	Parsley is anticancer and supports the immune system, tones bones, heals the nervous system, flushes water from the body (therefore supporting kidney function), and inhibits tumor formation. It is an excellent source of vitamin C, supports blood vessels, and protects from rheumatoid arthritis. It also lowers blood sugar. A study conducted at the University of Missouri found that a constituent found in parsley, celery, and other plants called "apigenin" decreases tumor size in an aggressive form of breast cancer.
Rosemary	Rosemary is rich in antioxidants and anti-inflammatory. It is anticancer. It improves circulation and digestion, enhances memory and concentration, provides neurological protection, prevents brain aging, and protects against macular degeneration.
Sage	Sage lowers blood sugar and cholesterol. It is a possible Alzheimer's treatment, improves brain function, and has antioxidant and anti-inflammatory properties.
Thyme	Thyme is antimicrobial. It lowers blood pressure, relieves coughs, and boosts mood and the immune system. It gets rid of pests (rats, mice, and others).
Natural unrefined salt or Himalayan salt	Natural unrefined salt or Himalayan salt helps stabilize irregular heart rate, regulates blood pressure, and extracts excess acidity from cells in the body (particularly brain cells). It balances blood sugar levels, clears lungs of excess mucus (particularly in asthma and cystic fibrosis), and clears sinus congestion. It is a natural antihistamine, regulates sleep, prevents muscle cramps, contributes to firm bones, helps prevent gout and gouty arthritis, is essential for maintaining sexual libido, and helps prevent varicose veins.

It supplies the body with over eighty essential mineral elements. Refined salt such as table salt has been stripped of all but two of these elements and contains harmful additives such as aluminum silicate, a toxic chemical found in a UK study to be the primary cause of neurological disorders such as Alzheimer's disease and Parkinson's disease.

Turmeric Turmeric is anti-inflammatory. It provides liver support, contains brain-protecting substances, boosts cognitive function, supports joint and muscle health, boosts detoxification, supports cardiovascular function, promotes healthy mood balance and radiant skin, and supports natural weight loss. Studies found that onions and turmeric synergistically work together to protect against cancer. Research shows that turmeric from Alleppey, India, contains nearly two times more curcumin (its active ingredient) than any other turmeric. One problem with curcumin is that it's not easily absorbed. Studies show that black pepper significantly enhances its bioavailability.

Note that most ground spices begin to fade in flavor and medicinal properties after a few months, so it's best to buy whole and grind as needed. Some herbs like cinnamon are somewhat tough, so you'll need a sturdy spice grinder or fine grater. If your only option is to buy ground spices, try to find high-quality ones made from organic spices.

Buy organic herbs and spices whenever possible. Herbs and spices that are either organic or wildcrafted are at their peak of maturity, and their concentration of active ingredients is highest, making them more effective than their counterparts. Organic herbs and spices are easy to find. They cost more, but not having pesticides, chemicals, and irradiation exposure makes them completely worth it.

Always add a label with the date you bought the spice on the day you bought them, and throw away whole spices if you haven't used them after two years and ground spices after six months.

TIPS TO INCORPORATE SPICES IN YOUR COOKING

The following are easy suggestions that will help you incorporate healing spices in your diet as preventive medicine:

- Flavor your milk or coffee with a pinch of nutmeg and cinnamon.
- Add whole cinnamon bark in soups or stews.
- Sprinkle cinnamon on fruits such as apples, bananas, melons, and oranges.
- Combine spices and use them as dry rubs for meats or fish:
    - Combine equal parts cinnamon, cardamom, and black pepper, and use as a rub for meats.
    - Grind coriander and rub it into meats or fish before cooking.
    - Rub ginger into the meat before grilling to help tenderize and add flavor.
- Add cinnamon to rice pilaf.
- Before sautéing vegetables or making stir-fry, sprinkle oil with turmeric.
- Add turmeric to fried onions.
- Use turmeric and ginger in lentil dishes.
- Blend turmeric in melted ghee and drizzle over cooked vegetables.
- Add a teaspoon of turmeric to a large pot of chicken noodle soup or homemade chili.
- Mix coriander seeds with peppercorns in your peppermill.
- Add whole or ground coriander seeds to stews, casseroles, marinades, vinaigrettes, and pickled dishes.

- Remember that fennel seeds naturally complement many foods from the Mediterranean diet, including tomatoes, olives, olive oil, basil, grilled meat, and seafood.
- Throw in extra fennel seeds the next time you make a sausage ragu.
- Add fennel seeds to fruit salads.

A FEW SAMPLE RECIPES TO WORK WITH HERBS AND SPICES

SPICED TEA

Put a quart of green, black, or any brewed tea into a pot. Add two cups of apple juice, and gently simmer with a sliced lemon and two cinnamon sticks for ten minutes.

SPICED OLIVES

Marinate for two hours (or up to two weeks) two cups of green olives in a half-cup of extra virgin olive oil and one teaspoon each of fennel seeds, dried oregano, and dried thyme.

HERB OIL

Herb oils are excellent in salads. They are good for sautés or on bread. Or they can be poured over sliced hard-boiled eggs. Use herbs such as basil, bay, dill, fennel, garlic, lemongrass, mint, oregano, rosemary, thyme, dried chilies or peppercorns, and the seeds of dill, fennel, cumin, or coriander. Make oil with a combination of herbs and spices or with a single herb. Use three to four tablespoons (or four to six sprigs) of fresh herbs and three cups of olive oil.

Method #1

Put the herbs into a sterilized jar and set aside. Heat oil until just warm and slowly pour over herbs. Once cool, strain into a sterilized bottle, cover, and label. Herb oils will keep for a week in the refrigerator.

Method #2

Place all of the herbs in a one-quart mason jar. Pour oil into a saucepan and heat to 195 degrees Fahrenheit. Pour the hot oils into the jar, and cover with a kitchen towel. Let stand overnight. Place cheesecloth over the top of the jar, and replace the outer rim of the lid. Invert and strain oil into the desired container.

BASIL SKIN TONER

This recipe is excellent for those with acne-prone skin. An antiseptic, basil helps clear acne-causing bacteria and improves skin circulation.

Crush three tablespoons of dried basil leaves and infuse them in one cup of boiling water. Let it sit for twenty minutes, strain out the leaves, put it in a spray bottle, and spritz your skin. Use a cotton ball to spread the toner gently around your face. Do this daily after cleansing. Discard after a week.

CINNAMON-CLOVE-GINGER BRONCHITIS REMEDY.

Mix one teaspoon each of ginger, cinnamon, and cloves in two cups of hot water. Decoct for twenty minutes. Add honey or stevia. Drink while hot. Combine these with other bronchitis remedies (such as herbal steams, tinctures, and so forth) for best effect. You may add a teaspoon of dried elderberries to improve taste and to create an even stronger remedy. Prolonged or severe bronchitis should be managed under physician supervision.

HOW TO MAKE HERBAL TEAS FROM SPICES

Cooking is not the only way you can take advantage of the medicinal properties of culinary herbs and spices. You can also make a delicious tea with them.

Use one tablespoon of dried herb or two tablespoons of fresh herb for each cup of water. There are two ways to make tea: infusions and decoctions.

- Infusions are for preparing teas containing the fragile parts of herbs and spices such as flowers, grasses, and leaves. Bring two cups of water to a boil, remove from heat, and place the spices in the water. You may put the herbs directly in the water or in a large muslin bag. Steep for at least twenty minutes.
- Decoction is used to break down more tenacious herb materials such as roots, bark, seeds, fruits, and nuts. Bring water to a boil, add the spices, lower heat to a gentle simmer, cover with a tight lid, and let brew for twenty minutes before turning off the heat. You may also soak tenacious herb materials overnight to soften them before simmering.

Be sure to strain before drinking. Strain and press down on the herbs to get all the tea out of the herbs.

As you can see, there are many health benefits to culinary herbs and spices, and it is straightforward to incorporate them into your life. I hope that the next time you are coming down with a cold, flu, or any other illness that this chapter has inspired you to reach into your spice rack instead of the medicine cabinet.

CHAPTER FIVE

The Role of the Environment in Health

Everything you see, hear, smell, taste, and touch is an environment. And those environments are either adding energy or draining energy.

—JIM BUNCH

An aspect of health that is often underestimated is the environment that we live and work in, including the people you spend the most time with. Your environment should be peaceful and clean and should invite you to want to be a part of it and to want to live or work there. The fact is, whatever is going on outside of you is also going on inside of you. If your external environments are chaotic and stressful, your internal environments will also be chaotic and stressful, and this can be harmful to your health or slow down your healing process.

Additionally, we are impacted and surrounded by different types of environments 24/7. Most people are unaware of the impact that those environments are having on their health and happiness. In fact, everything in our environment is either supporting us, giving us energy, and moving us closer to health or sabotaging, draining, and keeping us further away from health and our dreams.

The environment is stronger than willpower.
—Paramahansa Yogananda

According to the father of life coaching, Thomas Leonard, nine environments exist that are woven together and in constant interaction with us. These environments affect every aspect of us, and our environments reflect every part of us too. These environments are your support structure, and their quality can either support you emotionally, physically, or financially and are there for you if you fail, or they can bring you down and not allow you to grow and change. He further states it is essential that you design these environments in a way that they support and inspire your growth. Let's look now at the nine environments.

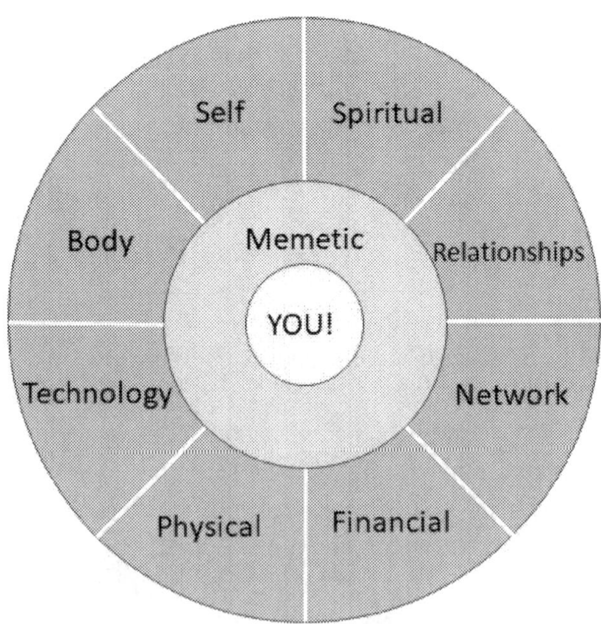

Figure. 3—The environments of you.

THE MEMETIC ENVIRONMENT

This includes your ideas, values, thoughts, beliefs, paradigms, and habits that are passed down from generation to generation. The memetic environment also is comprised of information and knowledge (books, classes, websites, magazines, television, and more). It is essential to take the time to think about how ideas from your society, friends, and family are impacting your health and desired results.

THE BODY ENVIRONMENT

The body environment includes your physical body such as hair, skin, nails, health, and energy. Being healthy and having strength, stamina, and overall well-being help you to be happy and to achieve your goals and desires. Building daily health habits, such as eating healthy and organic, exercising, and meditating are a great way to keep your body healthy.

Be mindful of environmental toxins that are all around us, from the food we eat and water we drink to the everyday products and energy we consume, such as endocrine disruptors found in plastic, pesticides found in food, and EMF found around the electronic devices that we use. In toxic doses, these toxins that can negatively affect your health are known to cause cancer, organ failure, and developmental, neurological, and reproductive problems.

THE SELF ENVIRONMENT

The self environment includes our feelings, emotions, values, passions, strengths, talents, personalities, and skills. The self environment reflects our inner resources and how we feel about ourselves to the outer world. Having a strong sense of self and self-love will support your growth.

THE TECHNOLOGY ENVIRONMENT

This includes social media, electronics, video conferencing, online networking, software, and hardware. Electronics include computers, tablets, phones, MP3 players, GPS systems, and so on. Having the necessary equipment and in good working condition to be able to maintain your personal and professional life flowing is essential to minimize stress.

THE SPIRITUAL ENVIRONMENT

The spiritual environment includes our connections to the universe or a higher power, or Spirit, and the connection we feel to our community and the rest of world. The source of your energy makes a difference in how you are going to experience your life. Energy from low vibrations such as the news or negative people may contribute to experiencing overwhelming feelings, clutter, addictions, control, anger, and so forth. On the other hand, high vibrations will bring about love and joy to your life. For this environment to be in balance, it is essential to include in your life spiritual practices that support you, such as meditation, laughter, gratitude, walking outdoors, being in nature, and so on.

THE RELATIONSHIP ENVIRONMENT

This environment includes the people who are in our lives on a daily basis, the closest to us, and with whom we have an intimate connection, such as family, close friends, close colleagues, coworkers, mentors, and so on. It is said that we are the average of the five people that are the closest to us. In other words, we become like the people we spend time with. Therefore, when it comes to spending time with people, choose wisely and make necessary changes. Additionally the people in your life act as a mirror to some part of yourself. Consequently, if you are always complaining about the people around you, it might be time to look at yourself and make changes there too.

THE NETWORK ENVIRONMENT

This environment is an expansion of the relationship environment. It includes your acquaintances, in other words, the people with whom you are on a first-name basis yet you may not have a deep connection with. The network environment comprises business associates, community organizations, and support groups. The goal of the network environment generally is to make available information for you and to build networks of people who can support you in enhancing both your business and personal life.

THE FINANCIAL ENVIRONMENT

The financial environment includes bills, credit cards, money, investments, insurance, stocks and bonds, and the people who support your economic well-being (accountants, financial planners, and stockbrokers). This environment also includes any tools, support services, or systems you use to achieve your financial goals such as computer programs, budgets, and banks. A balanced economic environment takes into consideration the relationship a person has with money and his or her beliefs about wealth, prosperity, and abundance.

THE PHYSICAL ENVIRONMENT

The physical environment includes our home, office, car, furnishings, artwork, and accessories. The physical environment provides visual clues to what is going on in our lives. Clutter, noise, and broken equipment can be a visual indication to look deeper at our thoughts and behaviors.

THE IMPORTANCE OF UPGRADING YOUR ENVIRONMENTS

Not having balanced and supportive environments is the reason people have a difficult time sticking with long-term changes. For example, people will make New Year's resolutions, and twenty days later, they're not working toward them. Or people will invest thousands of dollars to go to seminars, workshops, and books, but they're not achieving results. Some people will go as far as having open-heart surgery and then start eating junk food a few weeks after the surgery!

The fact is that we can't grow or function at a higher level while we are holding on to things, actions, or thoughts that are weighing us down. And an environment that is full of obstacles or is missing essential support will prevent us from growing and expanding and will make it difficult for us to succeed, regardless of what our goals are. Positive, well-designed environments are the key to your health and success.

You can't upgrade one environment and not it have it affect the others.
If you upgrade one environment it will send
a ripple through all the others.
—Jim Bunch

Consequently, when you become aware that everything, not just your physical space but also the people you talk to, the information you consume, the clothes you wear, and the food you eat are also part of your environment, you will develop a sense of appreciation and sensitivity of the impact of those environments to your health. And hopefully, you will make a conscious effort about upgrading the quality of those environments.

You can start with small changes. For example, you can declutter your bedroom or office, fix the garage door, clean out the garage, join a fitness club, hire a personal trainer or a life coach, buy a treadmill or weights, join a yoga class, move to a new area or city, take walks outside, spend more time with friends, stop spending time with negative people, cease watching the news, hire a financial planner, or read a positive book.

While it is true that our environments have a lot of impact over our feelings and actions, in the end, we have the ability and power to create environments that positively impact us. Your capacity to change is greater than you know. Therefore, regardless of what is going on in your mind and life, take action—even if you take small steps—in a positive and productive direction, and it will initiate the inspiration and transformation you have been waiting for.

PART TWO
Understanding the Problem

Health is a state of complete harmony of the body, mind and spirit. When one is free from physical disabilities and mental distractions, the gates of the soul open.

—B. K. S. IYENGAR

CHAPTER SIX

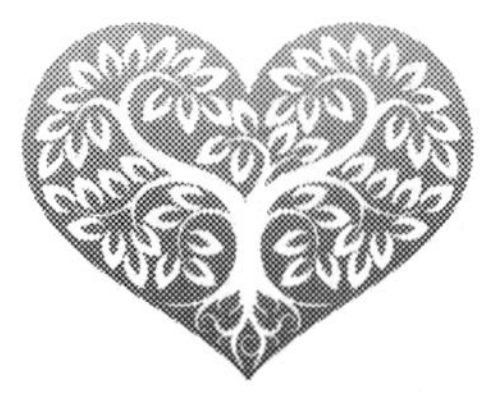

Who Gets Sick?

The simple truth is that happy people generally don't get sick.
—BERNIE SIEGEL

According to the CDC, chronic diseases and conditions—such as heart disease, stroke, cancer, type 2 diabetes, obesity, and arthritis—are among the most common of all health problems in the United States. And they predict that by the year 2030, the number of Americans living with a chronic disease will increase by 37 percent.[59] Moreover, the prevalence of both autoimmune diseases and allergies has been increasing since the 1950s, and the NIH estimates that one in five people are currently suffering from an autoimmune disorder.[60] That is 20 percent of the US population. That is a total of 65,313,660 people![61]

The most common symptom of an autoimmune disease and other chronic illness is inflammation. Inflammation is part of the body's immune response. It can be beneficial when, for example, your arm is hurt and tissues need to be repaired. Though, when inflammation sticks around more than necessary, it causes more harm than benefit. Many complex and interrelated factors can trigger chronic inflammation. However, the source can be narrow down to toxicity and deficiency due to emotional and physical stress, poor diet, and exposure to environmental toxins.

In the same way, it is a well-known fact that chronic diseases are primarily environmental and not genetic in origin.[62] In fact, the NIH reported that new studies have revealed that autoimmune diseases likely result from interactions between genetic and environmental factors.[60] According to the NIH, genetic predisposition accounts for approximately 30 percent of all autoimmune diseases. The remaining, 70 percent, is due to environmental factors, such as stress, toxic chemicals, dietary components, gut dysbiosis (imbalance or maladaptation), and infections.[63]

Additionally infections such as bacterial, viral, and parasitic infections, as well as some vaccines, are known to bring about and exacerbate autoimmune diseases.[64] Smoking has also been correlated with rheumatoid arthritis, systemic lupus erythematosus, thyroid disease, multiple sclerosis, and inflammatory bowel diseases.[65] Likewise, over the last few years, studies have expanded our previous knowledge of the gut and showed its wide-ranging importance and its potentials for triggering autoimmunity when dysbiosis occurs as a result of environmental factors.

Gut health is essential for your well-being. People with chronic illness, autoimmune disorders, and allergies in addition to dysbiosis often have a what is called a leaky gut, or "intestinal permeability," a condition caused by toxins and infections in which the lining of the small intestine becomes unhealthy and may have cracks or holes, causing undigested food particles, toxic waste products, and bacteria to "leak" through the intestines and go into the bloodstream. Consequently, this causes an autoimmune response in the body, including inflammatory and allergic reactions.

Moreover, the intestines will not produce the necessary enzymes for proper digestion. As a result, the body cannot absorb essential nutrients, which can lead to chronic illnesses, hormone imbalances, and a weakened immune system.

Autoimmunity happens over time, and often preclinical autoimmunity precedes clinical disease by many years. Initially, symptoms of autoimmune disorders are vague and include fatigue, low-grade fever, muscle and joint aches, and malaise. They usually progress and become debilitating with significant symptoms. Individuals are often seen by physicians only after their disease has become symptomatic, making it difficult to recognize the early events triggering the condition.[66]

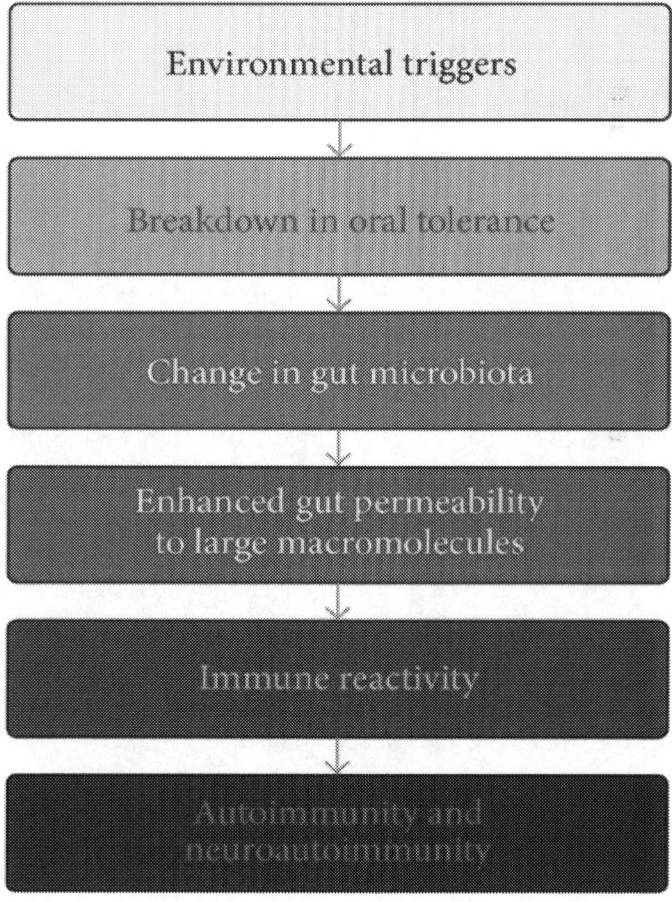

Figure 4—Mechanism for the awakening of autoimmunity and neuroautoimmunity by environmental triggers.[63]

Next, we will take a closer look at each one of the factors that may trigger autoimmune and chronic illnesses.

DIETARY DEFICIENCY AND TOXINS

Americans eat an average of 3,393 calories per day; it is almost double the number of the recommended daily calories. Unfortunately, even though Americans overeat, they are undernourished because of what they eat. The Standard American Diet, also known as the SAD diet, is mostly comprised of fattening foods that are devoid of nutrition. It lacks in vitamins, minerals, enzymes, and antioxidants while being high in refined sugar, refined grains, table (refined) salt, toxic protein, cholesterol, saturated fat, preservatives, and artificial flavors and coloring. These elements create chronic inflammation and consequently illness.

Likewise, toxicity starts in the soil of the plants we eat. Highly poisonous pesticides, fungicides, herbicides, and other chemicals used in commercial agriculture leave residues in our food even after washing. More importantly, since the emergence of GMOs, many of these chemicals are now a systemic part of the plant, as the seeds are stacked with herbicide-resistant traits.[67] Therefore they cannot be removed by washing. As covered in more detail in chapter 2, studies have demonstrated that glyphosate, an active ingredient in herbicides (pesticides), has been linked to many chronic illness and autoimmune disorders.

Additionally, chemicals are also added to our food when being processed. Chemical preservatives such as hydrogenated oils and high fructose corn syrup, amongst others, are added to extend the shelf life of a product to make them look more attractive and to enhance or replace natural flavors. These chemicals have been proven to increase the risk of inflammatory bowel diseases, metabolic disorders,[68] and cancer.[69]

Moreover, the prevalent use of food additives in commercial food—such as aspartame, MSG, sodium nitrate, saccharin, caffeine, fat substitutes, artificial colorings and flavorings, emulsifiers, flavor enhancers, thickening agents, trans fats, and unhealthily amounts of sugar, salt, and fat—provide no nutrition and are only in our food to improve appearance and taste, preserve, and lower production costs. Unfortunately these ingredients have also been linked to diseases, do not contain any nutritional value, and deliver toxicity the body is not always able to eliminate.

Furthermore, our society consumes too much sodium. In moderation, sodium is an essential mineral for your body to function correctly. However, most people's intake is so much that the kidneys have trouble keeping up with the excess in the bloodstream. As sodium accumulates, the body holds onto water to dilute the sodium. This increases both the volume of fluid and blood in the bloodstream. Increased blood volume means more work for the heart and more pressure on blood vessels. Over time, the extra work and stress can stiffen blood vessels, leading to high blood pressure, heart attack, stroke, and heart failure. There is also some indication that too much salt, in particular, table salt (refined), can be harmful to the bones and can damage the heart, aorta, and kidneys even without increasing blood pressure.

Another culprit of toxicity is the excess consumption of protein, in particular, in the form of animal protein. The ideal diet for humans should be primarily plant-based with minimal animal protein, such as the one described in chapter 2. Furthermore, eating animals raised on unhealthy food and treated with hormones, antibiotics, and synthetic growth promoters add to our level of toxicity. Additionally, long-term consumption of protein above the current recommended dietary allowance for adults (RDA: 0.8 g protein/kg body weight/day) has been linked with osteoporosis, kidney disease, calcium stones in the urinary tract, and some cancers.[70]

Also nowadays the media has been hyper-focusing on oxidative stress, which happens when you have too many free radicals in your body and not enough antioxidants to counterbalance them. Free radicals are created by emotional stress and toxic substances that are found in the food we eat, the drugs and medicines we take, the air we breathe, and the water we drink. These substances include fried foods, alcohol, tobacco smoke, pesticides, and air pollutants, amongst others.

These free radicals can cause damage to your cells, which can lead to cancer and other diseases. Consequently, due to the high media attention, many people are now taking antioxidant supplements and eating a large quaintly of foods that have high antioxidant content. One thing that may surprise you to know is that too many antioxidants can also lead to antioxidant stress. As with most things, trying to solve one issue by going overboard with therapies or supplements leads to a new set of problems. Like with everything in life, when taking antioxidants, moderation is the key.

Just like toxicity, an enemy of health is deficiency. Soil used in commercial agriculture uses fertilizers, which provide the soil nitrogen, phosphorous, and potassium. However, they do not offer fifty or more minerals and trace elements, which are essential to keep a fertile and healthy soil. As a result, this soil is weak and therefore produces deficient nutrient-poor plants. To make matters worse, these plants then get refined and processed, leaving us with minimal nutrients in the food we consume. As mentioned in chapter 3, organic foods have substantially more minerals, as much as 90 percent more compared with nonorganic foods. Therefore, to be healthy, it is recommended to eat organic whole foods whenever possible.

Equally essential to health is the consumption of an appropriate quantity of vitamins and minerals. An excess of vitamins and minerals, in particular, those that come from dietary supplements, can cause unwanted side effects. For example, an association has been made between high dietary calcium and increased prostate cancer[71] as well as kidney stones and kidney failure.[72] High intake of vitamin B_6 through food hasn't been shown to be harmful. However, in supplement form, too much vitamin B_6 also can cause a lack of muscle control or coordination of voluntary movements (ataxia); painful, disfiguring skin lesions; gastrointestinal symptoms such as heartburn and nausea; sensitivity to sunlight (photosensitivity); numbness; and reduced ability to sense pain or extreme temperatures. It has also been known to interfere with some medications such as chemotherapy drugs, barbiturates, anticonvulsants, and drugs for Parkinson's disease. Other side effects include but are not limited to excess zinc causing nausea, diarrhea, and stomach cramps and too much selenium leading to hair loss, gastrointestinal upset, fatigue, and mild nerve damage.

To function well, the human body needs thirteen essential vitamins and some fifty-two or so minerals, and it is critical to keep a good vitamin and mineral balance to keep up the body defenses. These minerals can easily be found in natural, fresh, organic vegetarian foods, such as whole grains, legumes, vegetables, and fruits.

Starting to see a pattern? Balance and moderation in the diet are vital to staying healthy. As you can see, even too much of a good thing can be detrimental to your health.

STRESS AND OTHER NEGATIVE EMOTIONS

Your emotional health also plays a role in the health of your body. As we covered in chapter 2, scientists are now discovering that changes in our consciousness produce changes in our bodies. Chronic stress and negative emotions such as worrying over mortgage payments, stressing over work, or keeping up with a packed schedule have an enormous negative impact on your health. Short-term stress can usually be dealt with, and as such, it does not adversely affect our bodies. However, when stress is chronic, it begins to disrupt the natural process of the body, and the immune system starts to become impaired. Cortisol, a hormone produced by the adrenals when you are under stress, negatively affects the digestive and immune system. Therefore, accumulated stress can lead to allosteric overload where serious health problems can result.

In fact, stress stimulates the immune system, which can help in immediate situations. This stimulation can help you avoid infections and heal wounds in case of an emergency. But over time, stress hormones will impair your immune system and reduce your body's response to foreign invaders. Therefore, people under chronic stress are more sensitive to viral illnesses like the flu and the common cold, as well as other infections. Also stress can lengthen the time it takes you to recover from a sickness or injury.

There is nothing wrong with experiencing negative thoughts and emotions like anger, resentment, and personal need. The problem is with habitual negative thinking that goes on day after day. It creates stress and causes an imbalance in your body that contributes to disease. Moreover, studies have linked chronic stress and negative emotions to headaches, infectious illness, cardiovascular disease, diabetes, asthma, gastric ulcers, obesity, erectile dysfunction, high blood pressure, and high cholesterol. Stress can also have an indirect effect on a person since people may use unhealthy coping strategies to reduce their stress, such as overeating, drinking, and smoking.

Other chronic negative emotions can also be harmful to your health. For example, anger and hatred are some of the most toxic emotions that we can experience. Feelings of rage and hatred do not only build up in the mind, but they also build up in the body, affecting the body's organs and natural processes, not to mention breeding even more negative emotions. The biological reason for this is epinephrine and norepinephrine constrict your blood vessels, making your heart work harder. They also increase the levels of glucose and fatty acids in your blood, which, when chronically elevated, damage your blood vessels and contribute to atherosclerosis. As with stress, short term, these emotions can usually be dealt with when they become chronic, and they cause harm to our bodies in the form of high blood pressure, stroke, stress, anxiety, headaches, and poor circulation and can impair the immune system.[62] Moreover, research has also shown that people who get angry easily tend to die sooner than their mellower peers.[63]

In addition to anger and hatred, other negative emotions such as depression, anxiety, and loneliness not only have broad health risks, such as a decrease in immune functioning, cardiovascular functioning, and cognitive functioning, it also increases a person's risk of heart disease and stroke by 29 and 32 percent, respectively.[73]

And if people have "already had a heart attack, these negative emotions (states of being) put them at increased risk for having another one," notes Donald Edmondson, director of the Center for Behavioral Cardiovascular Health at Columbia University Medical Center in New York City. Furthermore, extreme grief can also have a destructive impact on your health, and research confirms that, in the days after the loss of a loved one, your risk of experiencing a heart attack increases by twenty-one times. Likewise, according to Dr. Steven Standiford, chief of surgery at the Cancer Treatment Centers of America, unforgiveness is now classified in medical books as a disease and refusing to forgive causes people to get sick and keeps them that way.

Also according to Dr. Carsten Wrosch from Concordia University in Montreal, "Persistent *bitterness* may result in global feelings of anger and hostility that, when strong enough, could affect a person's physical health."[74] Moreover, research has shown that even a small amount of negative brain activity can lead to a weakened immune system, making you more prone to illness, and also lead to a heart attack or a stroke.

In the same way, studies at the Institute of HartMath demonstrate that changes in heart-rhythm patterns are clearly reflected when an individual is experiencing positive or negative emotions. For example, their research shows that sustained positive feelings are associated with a noticeably coherent, smooth, and balanced heart-rhythm pattern. In contrast, negative emotions are reflected by a jagged, erratic pattern.[75]

THE FIVE ELEMENTS AND THE EMOTIONS

Similarly, from the Eastern medicine perspective, extreme emotions can affect our bodies. In TCM, the belief is that each emotion influences a specific organ; likewise each organ gives rise to a feeling. Under normal conditions, this relationship helps a person respond to an event. Unfortunately, as we get older and encounter more stress in our daily lives, negative emotions such as fear, anger, cruelty, impatience, worry, sadness, and grief often predominate in our lives.

When these feelings are excessive or underdeveloped, the body will eventually get sick. Additionally, the extreme up-and-down seesaw effect of emotions (positive or negative) can subsequently compromise our health. Therefore, one of the keys to good health is to become aware how these emotions affect our health and to learn to transform the negative emotions into positive virtues such as love, gentleness, kindness, respect, honesty, fairness, justice, and righteousness.

This table describes the seven emotions and their influence on the human body according to the five element theory.

Element	Organ	Emotion	Organ-Emotion Influence on the Body
Fire	Heart	Joy	Excessive joy (mania) consumes heart energy, leading to a deficiency in heart energy. It also relaxes the heart so it cannot function correctly.
Wood	Liver	Anger	Excessive anger consumes liver energy, leading to a deficiency of liver energy. It also rises to the head, creating headaches, high blood pressure, and potentially strokes.

Element	Organ	Emotion	Organ-Emotion Influence on the Body
Metal	Lungs	Worry and Sadness	Excessive worry and sadness consumes lung energy, leading to deficient lung energy. This can cause abdominal pain and swelling
Earth	Spleen	Thought	Excessive thinking uses up spleen energy, which can cause deficient spleen energy and causes the congestion of the spleen
Water	Kidneys	Fear and Shock	Excessive fear and shock consume kidney energy, leading to a deficiency of kidney energy. Fear also moves energy downward, causing lower body problems and kidney issues. Shock causes chaos in the kidneys and makes them inefficient.

As described in chapter 3, in the five element theory, an imbalance of the organs can also give rise to emotions, and the key to healing the body is by balancing the elements. For example, excessive anger can arise from a stagnant liver (or contribute to it), and the inability to express anger can come from a weak liver system. Likewise, the opposite is true. we can affect an organ by experiencing an emotion in excess. For example, constant anger can cause a liver imbalance such as stagnation or weakness.

Another important concept in Chinese medicine that is worth considering when looking at chronic illness and autoimmune disorders is the fundamental role that the spleen plays in digestion. It is paired with the stomach, and together they are responsible for the absorption and distribution of food and nutrients throughout our bodies. The spleen extracts energy (qi) from the food we eat to build immunity, to keep things moving freely for the proper functioning of the other organs, and to help to regulate emotions.

It is very common in our culture to have a spleen deficiency. Many things can cause a deficiency of spleen qi. However, a poor diet of mostly refined, highly processed foods where the body is not receiving enough nourishment is one of the main reasons. Another cause is our hectic lifestyles and excess of worry and overthinking, as well as having a hard time just slowing down our thoughts. In brief, a deficiency of the spleen leads to stagnation and consequently illness.

In short, both traditional medicine and science support the fact that our thoughts and feelings play a distinct role in our experience of physical pain and can cause the development of chronic disease. Moreover, in the same way as with food, balance and moderation of emotions are vital to staying healthy, and even too much of a good thing, such in the case as extreme joy (mania), can be detrimental to your health.

ENVIRONMENTAL TOXINS

Many everyday environmental factors such as toxins and endocrine disruptors have been linked to the increase in the last few decades of asthma, allergies, autoimmune disorders, dramatic changes in the activity, and balance of the immune system and other inflammatory reactions.

Environmental toxins can be both human-made and naturally occurring, and in toxic doses, they can negatively affect your health. They are known to cause cancer, organ failure, and developmental, neurological, and reproductive problems.[76] Let's review them.

Endocrine disruptors imitate the action of steroid hormones in the body and have promoted endocrine and reproductive disorders such as obesity, infertility, aggressive behavior, early onset of puberty, hormone-dependent cancers (prostate and breast), thyroid dysfunction, lower testosterone levels, and sperm production.

Toxins are found in the air, water, and soil, and many have undesirable effects on human health such as allergies, asthma, headaches, fatigue, insomnia, dizziness, hand tremors, other neurological symptoms, chronic inflammatory diseases, and a negative impact on immune modulation.

Environmental toxins are all around us, from the air we breathe, the food we eat, water we drink, and to the everyday products and energy we consume, for example:

- BPA is found in plastic bottles.
- Phthalates are found in bottles, shampoo, cosmetics, lotions, nail polish, and deodorant.
- Pesticides are found in nonorganic foods.
- Lead (Pb) is found in old paint and old pipes.
- Mercury is found most commonly as a by-product of pollution and a dietary source often found in seafood, but it can also come from livestock-fed contaminated fishmeal and plants grown in contaminated soil, pesticides, protein powder, and fish oil.
- Radon can be released from building materials and water wells, and it is in nearly all soils and can get to your home through cracks in floors, walls, and foundations.
- Formaldehyde is used in building materials and the manufacture of many household products such as press-wood, glues and adhesives, permanent press fabrics, cigarette smoke, and fuel-burning appliances. It is also used as an industrial fungicide, germicide, and disinfectant.
- Benzene, a petrochemical, is found in tobacco smoke, gasoline, pesticides, synthetic fibers, plastics, inks, oils, detergents, and dryer sheets.
- Cadmium is found in industrial workplaces, plant soils, cigarette smoke, and our drinking water.[77]
- Carbon monoxide is found in diesel and other exhaust fumes, smoke from fires, and nonelectric heaters.
- Fluoride, one of the main routes through which people can be exposed, is in our drinking water[78] and toothpaste.
- Chlorine is also found in our water and household cleaning products.

- Many studies have documented an autoimmune reaction and immunological dysfunction in patients with silicone breast implants. These immune abnormalities and symptoms are reversible upon removal of the breast implants (in 50 to 70 percent of cases).[79]
- Virtually all antibiotics and other medications (drugs) are toxic but sometimes necessary. Use them wisely.
- Electromagnetic fields (EMF) is the latest addition to environmental pollution. It is found around electronic devices, such as cordless phones, hair dryers, vacuums, refrigerators, microwave ovens, irons, lighting circuits, dimmer switches, electric blankets, electric razors, electric toothbrushes, Wi-Fi, computers, fluorescent or halogen lighting, fax machines, photocopiers, scanners, cell phones, power lines, transformers, electrical substations, and cell phone towers.

TOXINS FROM YOUR MEMETIC AND RELATIONSHIP ENVIRONMENTS

As covered in the last chapter, your environment is not just your physical space, the clothes you wear, and the food you eat, but it also includes the people you spend time with and the information you consume. Therefore, the quality of those environments is equally essential to your health.

Let's start with negative people. Negative people bring down your mood and impact your health with their pessimism, anxiety, and a general sense of distrust. Be aware that negativity is highly contagious and constant exposure to negativity can affect your level of positivity, leading you to either become negative, reserved, anxious, and distrustful or to become indifferent, uncaring, or even mean toward the negative person.

Moreover, research in the field of neuroscience has demonstrated that others can have an effect on the physical structure of our brain. This new study published in the journal *Nature Neuroscience* shows that stress conveyed to you by others may affect your brain in the same way as your own stress does (mirror neurons).

Similarly, the human heart emits the most energetic electromagnetic field in our body, and the quality of this field changes according to our emotions. This field envelops the entire body, and it can measure up to several feet away from the human body. Therefore, you are in constant contact with the electromagnetic field of the people that are near you. Positive emotions, as covered in chapter 2, create physiological benefits in your body, such as boosting your immune system and coherent heart-rhythm.

On the other hand, experiencing negative emotions, as seen earlier in this chapter, can create a nervous system and heart chaos and that not only impact our health but the health of those around our electromagnetic field. "We are fundamentally and deeply connected with each other and the planet itself, and what we do individually really does count and matters," states Rolin McCratey, PhD, director of research at the HeartMath Institute.

Furthermore, due to the phenomena of emotional contagion, negative emotions exert a more powerful effect in social situations than positive ones. "Anger and resentment are the most contagious of emotions," says Dr. Steven Stosny, expert in anger management in relationships. He further states,

> If you are near a resentful or angry person, you are more prone to become resentful or angry yourself. If one driver engages in angry gestures and takes on the facial expressions of hostility, surrounding drivers will unconsciously imitate the behavior—resulting in an escalation of anger and resentment in all the drivers. Added to this, the drivers are now more easily startled because of the outpouring of adrenaline accompanying their anger. The result is a temper tantrum that can easily escalate into road rage.

Equally important to how negative people affect us is how the emotional content of the news, films, books, and television programs impact our psychological health. According to Graham C. L. Davey, PhD, they can do this by directly affecting our mood, and our mood can then change many aspects of our thinking and behavior. For this reason, not only will they make you sad and anxious, they are also likely to exacerbate your own personal worries and anxieties.[80]

PART THREE

The Solution
A Multidimensional Health Program

"Health is a state of complete harmony of the body, mind and spirit. When one is free from physical disabilities and mental distractions, the gates of the soul open."

—B. K. S. IYENGAR

CHAPTER SEVEN

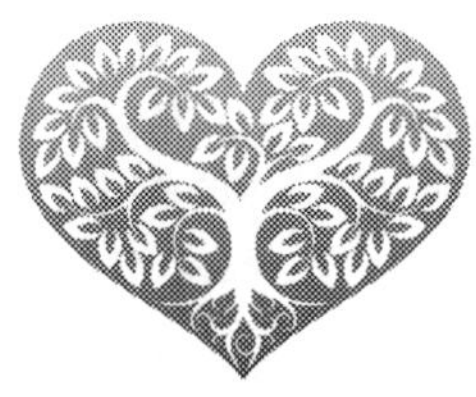

How to Heal and Prevent Illness

The greatest medicine of all if to teach people how not to need it.
—HIPPOCRATES

The good news is that, by taking some simple and inexpensive measures, such as consuming high-quality herbal supplements and watching what you eat and think, chronic and autoimmune disorders are preventable and can be treated and, in many cases, reversed. It sounds too simple to be true but is not. Traditional medicine has successfully applied this approach for centuries, and millions of people have healed using this approach, such is the case as Kellie Alderton, who healed herself from MS using traditional medicine. This is her story.

> At the age of seventeen (1988), I was diagnosed with multiple sclerosis. I grew up in a home with a very controlling and mentally abusive parent. Consequently I was constantly under a lot of stress, and I had a poor diet. I also had many bouts of strep throat and tonsillitis. We also had a home full of chemicals. My dad was all

> about having the greenest yard and cleanest (bleached) pool. It was a perfect storm for illness.
>
> After my diagnosis, I went for thirteen years on the MS roller coaster with conventional medicine MS therapies that kept me sick, consistent relapses, and with no quality of life. Finally in 2001, I turned to holistic and natural therapies to heal and never looked back. Diet, supplements, and healing the mind and spirit were the key for me to beating MS. I believe these therapies saved my life! Now after years of studying nutrition, healing, and personal development, I'm convinced we can heal our bodies naturally if we focus on the mind-body-spirit connection and being healthy and whole in each of those areas. I'm living symptom-free now, healthy, and strong for over fourteen years.

You can read more about Kellie's journey to health in her book, *Waking Up from MS—My Journey to Health, Healing, and Living Symptom-Free.*

Just like Kellie, millions of people all over the world are using this multidimensional approach to health. In fact, up to 90 percent of the population in Africa and 70 percent of the population in India relies on traditional medicine to help meet their health-care needs.[1] In China, traditional medicine accounts for around 40 percent of all health care administered, and more than 90 percent of general hospitals in China have units for holistic medicine.[81]

Furthermore, the use of traditional medicine is not limited to developing countries. In the United States in 2012, about 38 percent of adults and 12 percent of children were using some form of traditional medicine.[82] Additionally, a survey conducted in Hong Kong in 2003 reported that 40 percent of the subjects surveyed showed significant faith in traditional medicine compared with Western medicine.[83]

In the same way, as mentioned in earlier chapters of this book, it is scientifically proven that our bodies respond to how we think and feel, and each of our thoughts and feelings create a cascade of biochemicals in our body. Each experience produces a positive or negative change in our cells, consequently in our health. Therefore, it is not enough to eat well and do exercise. Instead health is something that needs to be looked at in three areas: emotions (awareness), body, and spirit.

Without this multidimensional approach, it will be difficult to find the level of balance needed to live a healthy life. Note that this integrative approach to health does not exclude conventional medicine. There is a time and a place for conventional medicine, for example, if you have a heart attack, a car accident, or internal bleeding, as well as times where we need lab work or imaging done, amongst many other situations.

Western medicine has also provided us with fantastic scientific research that validates and supports traditional medicine theories and practices. However, an integrative approach to health encourages prevention and awareness (emotions) as a primary element and a vital key to health, followed by exercise and food. The following integrative health pyramid shows the hierarchy of the preferred treatment approach.

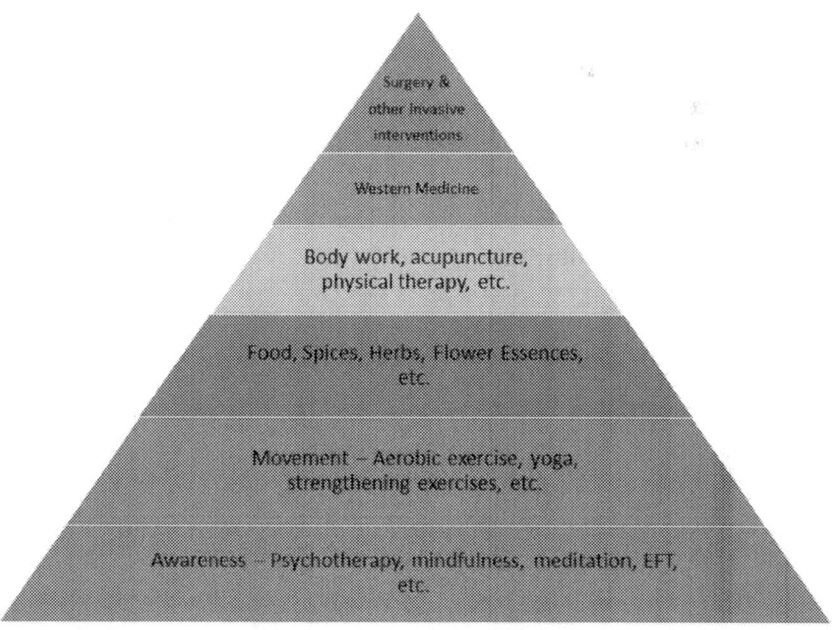

Figure 5—Integrative health pyramid.

As you can see, the first three base elements in the pyramid are mostly lifestyle actions such as proper nutrition, exercise, adequate rest, and emotional and spiritual balance as well as the emphasis on preventing disease and maintaining health. These elements encourage and empower an individual to participate in and take responsibility for his or her health.

The power to heal is within you. The health program covered in this book will only work if you take 100 percent responsibility for your health and your life. No more blaming our genes, age, pesticides, mercury retrograde, astrological sign, cell towers, and so on. Taking responsibility for your health is not about making you feel bad, guilt, or punishment. Instead it is about empowerment and taking control of your health. There is no need to judge or criticize yourself for your current health status. Know that you are always doing the best you can with the limited awareness that you have at the moment.

However, until you can honestly accept and say, "I have a choice in my health and how I live my life. I am in this place now because of the choices I've made in the past," you will not be able to say, "I will make different choices." You got yourself consciously or unconsciously into your current health situation, and you can get out of it by taking responsibility for your life and making the changes needed to live a healthy life, as Jim Rohn said, "You can't hire someone else to do push-ups for you."

Remember, you are your choices. You and only you can heal yourself, according to Louise Hay, motivational author and the founder of Hay House, if you are willing to do the work. Almost any disorder can heal, and she suggests that it is impossible to do inner work without improving the quality of your life. More importantly, "When people change the new personality often does not need the old disease, so their body heals," she often said.

For this reason, when I work with clients, I dedicate time to learn about the habits that may have brought them to their current health condition, and we work on building new practices that will guarantee not only a successful recovery but prevent future diseases. My approach is multidimensional, and I take into consideration physical symptoms as well as emotions and their environments as I personalize their health plan.

Nevertheless, even if you do not have a custom-designed health plan, there is a core protocol that almost anyone can follow to heal autoimmune disorders and chronic illnesses. Next, I share with you the core protocol that I use and adapt to each of my client's needs. This protocol includes but is not limited to:

1. Gently cleanse while nourishing the body.
2. Restore gut health and support the immune system.
3. Minimize environmental toxins.
4. Improve emotional health and support the nervous system and adrenals.

The rest of this section will elaborate in detail each item in this protocol so you can apply it to your life. Don't get overwhelmed with all the information provided in the following section, part four of this book, I will take you through an easy step-by-step process to implement everything you learn in this book.

CHAPTER EIGHT

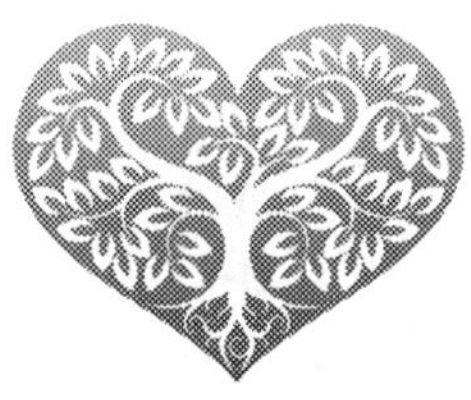

Gently Clear Toxins While Nourishing

Every time you either eat or drink, you are either feeding disease or fighting it.

—HEATHER MORGAN, MS, NLC

As mentioned in previous chapters, many symptoms of chronic illness and autoimmune disorders can be linked to an impaired digestive and detoxification system. Proper nutrition, a well-functioning digestive, and detoxification system are essential to maintain a healthy weight, reduce your risk of chronic diseases, and promote your overall health. Therefore, to improve your health, no matter what condition you have, you will need to nourish and gently cleanse your body with food and herbs first.

> Several years ago, I was diagnosed with three uterine fibroids. One of them was three centimeters long. My doctor thought that the best approach for me was to surgically remove them. However, I knew that the reason I had them was due to excess estrogen in my body caused by environmental toxins such as pesticides. So against

> doctors' orders, I made the decision to treat them with natural medicine. First, I went back to eating healthy and following the diet outlined in chapter 9. In particular, I was strict about not eating anything that was not organic because I knew pesticides are estrogen disruptors. Then I designed an herbal formula with liver detox and hormone-balancing herbs.
>
> Per my doctor's request, after two months of this regimen, I went back to get an ultrasound. The large polyp was still there but had changed shape. It was thinner now. My doctor insisted that I should have surgery because, in her opinion, natural medicine did not work. I refused because, to me, progress was being made. And again, against doctors' orders, I continued my regimen.
>
> Two months later, I had another ultrasound, and the polyps were completely gone. My doctor was surprised and could not believe the ultrasound. When I asked her if she believed now that natural medicine worked, she said, "No, this was just a coincidence. Sometimes this type of things just happens."

My story is common occurrence. In general, people in the West are deficient or weak due to toxin overload and lack of nourishment. (See chapter 6 for more details.) Therefore, it is essential that we nourish the body while we are doing a cleanse. Otherwise, depending on your level of health, cleansing without nourishing may put too much strain on your body, consequently making it weaker and hindering recovery. Mainly for people suffering from a digestive or an autoimmune disorder, supplementation and easily digested foods, such as congee and soups are necessary to combat nutrient loss through diarrhea, pain, and nausea. Additionally, certain times of the year are more suitable for cleansing, such as early spring (March or April). However, if you are already suffering from a chronic or autoimmune disease, there is no time like the present to start this program.

CLEANSING WITH FOODS

The following foods nourish the body while helping you detoxify:

1. Consume green plants that clean and renew the liver such as:

    a. Chlorella regenerates cells and organs.

    b. Wild blue-green algae is highly cleansing yet nurturing to the liver.

    c. Seaweeds are also cleansing and restore the liver and gallbladder.

    d. Eat fruits that contain phytochemicals and antioxidants, such as berries, pomegranate, and grape. Watch your fruit intake if you are a diabetic.

    e. Lemon and lime can be squeezed into water or used in food preparation on a daily basis.

    f. Cilantro gently removes toxins from the body. It removes arsenic, cadmium, aluminum, lead, and mercury in our tissues.

    g. Basil is alkalizing, supports liver function, and detoxifies the body.

2. Incorporate into your diet sharper-tasting bitter greens like arugula, kale, watercress, mustard, and dandelion greens. They are bitter leafy greens packed with nutrition and alkaline-forming, and they have a detoxifying effect on the body.

3. Complex Carbohydrates are essential for proper peristalsis (bowel movement) to take place. The body needs to have adequate amounts of complex carbohydrates in the form of vegetables, fruits, legumes, and whole grains. These foods are high in fiber. Including more fiber in your diet provides the bowel more material to work with when eliminating waste from your body, and it will require less time to transit time through the body. On the other hand, refined carbohydrates form soft stools which are more difficult for the bowel to move along and eliminate. Refined carbohydrates create a white sticky mass within the gut that hinders the peristaltic action of the digestive tract, causing waste to stagnate and consequently prolonging elimination time.

4. The pungent taste can be found in numerous spices and vegetables, such as chili peppers, garlic, onions, mustard, turnips, scallions, daikon

radish, black radish, horseradish, red radish, wasabi, black pepper, ginger, and cayenne.

The difference between spicy and pungent is negligible. The pungent taste warms the body, cleanses the mouth, clarifies the sense organs, enhances other flavors, and improves digestion, absorption, and elimination. Additionally the pungent taste clears congested sinuses, promotes sweating and detoxification, helps to discharge gas, and improves circulation. It is stimulating, invigorating, and penetrating, and it removes moisture, stagnation, and congestion. It also increases circulation, removes toxins, cleanses the blood and the muscles, reduces cholesterol, and clears blockages.

You should not limit your diet just to these foods. It is also not recommended to overeat them. Instead follow the guidelines in chapter 3 for the optimum ratios of carbohydrates, vegetables, and proteins, and add the recommended foods from this list to your meals.

CLEANSING WITH THE HELP OF HERBS

Cleansing and liver support herbs taken daily gently accelerate the detoxifying process while supporting the liver and kidneys in flushing ingested and environmental toxins from the body. These herbs include but are not limited to:

- Dandelion has a diuretic effect, allowing the liver and kidneys to eliminate toxins faster. It also helps strengthen the immune system, balance blood sugar levels, relieve heartburn, and soothe digestive issues.
- Burdock, an alterative, purifies the blood, improves liver function, and promotes the production of bile, which the liver secretes, assisting the body to excrete waste products from the blood. Burdock also is a diuretic. Therefore, it aids in eliminating excess water by increasing urine output, which helps the kidneys remove toxins. Other uses include reduced cell mutation. Consequently it is anticancer and antitumor. It is anti-inflammatory, antioxidant, and antibacterial.

- Red clover is an excellent blood purifier that gradually cleanses the bloodstream and corrects deficiencies in the circulatory system. It has been shown to thin the blood and reduce the possibility of blood clots and arterial plaques. It is anticancer. Estrogenic, it has been used to treat symptoms of PMS and menopause, promote breast health, and prevent osteoporosis.

- Milk thistle helps to detoxify the liver and encourages the elimination of toxic waste from the colon. Milk thistle is also anti-inflammatory and is thought to be able to support healthy digestive function by promoting enzyme formation, increasing bile production, and soothing the mucous membranes throughout the body.

- Sassafras is a diuretic, thus eliminating excess toxins, salts, and fats from the body. Sassafras is also used to eliminate colds, boost kidney health, relieve pain, prevent cancer, boost the immune system, soothe inflammation, reduce menstruation pain, and increase energy. Its antiseptic properties help protect dental health.

- Yellow dock is a blood purifier and general detoxifier, in particular for the liver. Yellow dock root stimulates bile production, which helps digestion of fats. It also encourages bowel movements to help eliminate lingering waste from your intestinal tract. It is also a diuretic; therefore, it increases the frequency of urination to assist in toxin elimination.

- Schizandra improves liver function, digestive health, and the ability to remove waste from the body. Schizandra also boosts antioxidant activity and improves circulation and digestion. It is also anti-inflammatory and immune boosting and supports adrenal function.

- Lavender essential oil assists in the breakdown of toxic materials from environmental toxins in the lymph, liver, and viscera. It also helps break down hydrogenated oils, trans- fats, and synthetic polymers (from poor-quality deep-fried oils, shortening, and margarine).[54]

WATER

Water is crucial to any cleansing program for diluting and eliminating accumulations. Drink eight to ten glasses a day at least. However, it is recommended you drink half your body weight in ounces. For instance, if you weigh two hundred pounds, you will need to drink one hundred ounces of water per day. Do not drink with meals. Instead drink thirty minutes before or after meals.

DEEP BREATHING IS CLEANSING AND GOOD FOR YOUR HEALTH

Breathing promotes the creation of white blood cells. Every time you inhale, your lungs fill with oxygen, and from there oxygen, gets transported throughout your body, including the organs of detoxification such as lymphatic system, kidneys, and colon. At the same time, when we exhale, we eliminate our body's waste in the form of carbon dioxide. Consequently, when we practice deep rhythmic breathing, we take in even more oxygen to clean the body, and when we exhale deeply, we eliminate more waste.

However, most of us are unaware that we are breathing shallowly throughout the day, resulting in minimal breath into our lungs. Shallow breathing can also be triggered by anxiety, stress, and bad posture, amongst many other things, leading to side effects that include fatigue and decreased tissue function. Moreover, if you aren't breathing deeply or moving on a regular basis, your lymphatic fluids become stagnant, and this blocks the system from adequately eliminating waste. A poorly functioning lymphatic system can lead to high blood pressure, heart problems, weight gain, fatigue, and inflammation.

Therefore, to assist your body in the detoxification process, you must take deep breaths as often as possible throughout the day. However, if you have a hectic lifestyle, you can practice the following deep breathing exercise first thing in the morning when you wake up and at the end of the day before going to bed.

1. Place the tip of your tongue against the ridge behind your upper teeth and exhale completely through your mouth so you make a whoosh sound.

2. Close your mouth and inhale deeply through your nose for a count of four, hold your breath for seven counts, and then exhale through your mouth for a count of eight.

3. Repeat three times.

CHAPTER NINE

The Diet

One of the biggest tragedies of human civilization is the precedence of chemical therapy over nutrition. It's a substitution of artificial therapy over nature, of poisons over food, in which we are feeding people poisons trying to correct the reactions of starvation.

—DR. ROYAL LEE

I believe that no one diet fits all. That is why, in my practice, I customized my clients' diets based on their condition, constitution, personality, and emotional issues that they may be experiencing. Yes! You read correctly. You can choose foods that will benefit you based on your makeup and emotions. (See chapter 3 for more details.) This concept is based on Eastern medicine where one of the fundamental principles is that we should eat according to who we are. Therefore, there is no such thing as a universal right diet. Instead each person will have various constitution and needs, consequently different nutritional needs. However, the following is a base diet that anyone regardless of his or her health condition can benefit from.

You can add and remove foods to this diet based on your individual needs. In particular, incorporate the cleansing foods listed in chapter 8 as well as foods from the five element table listed in chapter 1. Select foods from the element that you may think you have an imbalance or an element that you feel you may be deficient. For example, if you are having problems letting go of the past or lung issues (metal element), to increase the presence of metal energy, you might eat more rice, pungent foods, and contracted root vegetables.

Similarly, for proper nutritional content and for helping to cleanse the liver, you should incorporate a balance of all flavors (salty, sweet, sour, and bitter) and colors in your diet. Likewise, buy organic produce whenever possible to limit your exposure to pesticide, GMOs, and other environmental toxins. Additionally, organic fruits and vegetables are considerably more nutritious than nonorganic.

WHAT TO EAT?

You will want to focus on eating a *nutrient-dense* diet. This is important because when the body is weak and malnourished, it does not have the strength and capacity to bring about health and symptom relief. As covered in chapter 6, to function well, the human body needs some fifty-two or so minerals, and it is essential to keep a proper mineral balance to keep up the body's defenses. These minerals can be found in natural, fresh, organic vegetarian foods, such as whole grains, legumes, vegetables, and fruits. Incorporate these into your diet.

Until sufficient improvement has been made, take care to prepare meals that are easier to digest. For example, soups, vegetable smoothies, and juices made with fresh food (not frozen), none-gluten protein smoothies, and stews are all great options. Furthermore, it is important to eat foods that support the spleen. From the Chinese medicine perspective, to keep the spleen healthy, it is important to eat as mindfully as possible. (See chapter 3 for details.)

The spleen also likes warm foods. So you will want to incorporate foods and spices that are warming in nature or at least neutral to help build the spleen's energy, for example, spices, black pepper, ginger, nutmeg, cinnamon, fennel, and garlic. The flavor associated with the spleen is sweet, such as pumpkin, yam, black beans, garbanzo beans, carrot, parsnip, squash, peas, sweet potato, onion, leek, and fennel. Cold and raw foods should be minimized as it is believed they weaken digestion. Also foods that are cold in temperature take more energy for the spleen to digest.

Some examples of what to eat to nourish your body while helping you detoxify are:

- To settle down autoimmune response, include foods high in *magnesium* in your diet.
- Eat plenty of soups. Soups are full of nutrients and easier to digest.
- One of the best foods to support the spleen is cooked brown rice, often eaten in the form of congee. (See recipe in chapter 3.)
- Lemon water is very cleansing and supportive to the liver.
- Soy-free Miso soup. Miso is alkaline-forming and loaded with probiotic cultures. It has been used traditionally to help health conditions, such as fatigue, to regulate digestive and intestinal functions, protect against gastric ulcers, decrease cholesterol and blood pressure levels, prevent inflammation, and lower the risk for diseases associated with lifestyle and environmental factors, like cancers and heart disease. If you are not sensitive to soy, you can eat regular miso soup.
- Aim for two servings of beets per day. They are rich in antioxidants and anti-inflammatory. They support detoxification and build your blood.
- Eat anti-inflammatory, detoxifying, and nutrient-dense foods. See foods such as leafy greens, radishes, carrots, brussels sprout, sprouts, seedlings, chlorophyll, turmeric, garlic, onions, and other medicinal spices. (See chapter 8 for complete list.)
- Cruciferous vegetables contain nutrients that help support the liver's detoxification. Cabbage, broccoli, cauliflower, kale, and turnips are crucifers.
- Cilantro and fiber excrete toxins and excess hormones.

- Green smoothies or juices should be made of primarily green vegetables with a little fruit, like green apple, for flavor.
- Fermented foods are full of probiotics that support gut and the detox process.
- Berries contain phytonutrients and antioxidants and are low in glycemic index.
- Seaweeds are a rich source of vitamins, including vitamin A, C, D, E, and K. They are also a great source of minerals such as potassium and iodine. Despite being low in fat, some species of seaweed contain DHA and omega-3. Blue or green Algae is a complete food source (provides our daily nutritional requirements).
- Avocados are highly nutritious and contain 20 different vitamins and minerals, including a high content of potassium. Therefore, they promote the opening and expansion of the cells in our bodies.
- Eat nuts and other good fats in moderation. See the food pyramid in chapter 3 for daily proportions. Nuts contain some important essential vitamins and minerals, such as vitamin A, iron, B vitamins, manganese, and folate, as well as protein, healthy fats, and antioxidants. Soak them for an hour or two before cooking or eating them.
- Glands, in general, require-high quality protein and fat to function correctly. Therefore, it will significantly benefit your body to increase your intake of *Omega-3 fatty acids* in the form of fish or seed oil, such as flax and chia seed.
- Incorporate in your food oils such as olive, coconut, avocado, sesame, safflower, rice bran, and flaxseed. Each oil has different qualities and is better for different uses. Some are best used for baking, like coconut oil. Some are best for frying, like avocado, peanut and coconut oils, and some work best in salad dressings like olive and sesame oils. Select the oil according to its health benefits and the needs of your recipe.
- If you are taking nutritional supplements, whenever possible consume those produced from whole foods, such as nutritional

yeasts, seaweed, algae, or vitamin and mineral supplements made with food as in the following brands: *Health Force Nutritionals, New Chapter, Nature's Plus, Garden of Life and Natural Vitality* to name a few.

You should not limit your diet just to these foods. Instead eat a variety of foods and follow the guidelines in chapter 3 for the optimum ratios of carbohydrates, vegetables, and proteins, and to make sure you eat the recommended foods during the week.

HOW TO EAT?

This table outlines a sample diet plan to follow for this program. However, you may adjust accordingly to your personal schedule and lifestyle. The diet will work as long as you incorporate all the elements in the table below and the food recommendations made in this book (chapters 3, 8, and 9).

Time	Food
7:00 a.m. or when you wake up	Drink a cup of Miso soup or lemon water. Squeeze half a lemon in a cup of water; add honey or maple syrup to taste.
8:00 a.m. or your usual breakfast time	*Breakfast smoothie:* Mix one cup of mixed greens, one carrot, half an avocado (or another source of good fat such as almonds or cashews soaked overnight), one stick of celery, one cucumber, a few basil leaves, one cup coconut milk, one beet, and one scoop of pea protein powder. This is meant to be a savory smoothie. Therefore, if you would like to improve the taste, you can add lemon. If you prefer a sweeter flavor then, then add one-half or one cup of mix berries. To support the spleen, try to use fresh ingredients as much as possible instead of frozen (warmer). Additionally fresh ingredients have more life force and are more nutritious.
10:00 a.m.	Make a green smoothie of your choice, primarily made of green vegetables with a little fruit, like green apple, for sweetness

12:00 p.m.	Incorporate into your lunch soups, good fats, fiber, grains (non-glutenous grains if you are gluten intolerant), legumes, vegetables, and clean animal protein, if desired, Congee can be eaten too.
3:00 p.m.	Make nutritive herbal tea with herbs such as nettles, oats, and alfalfa. Or for chai latte, mix one tablespoon of maca powder (which reishi or astragalus can replace), one tea bag of caffeine-free chai, and one cup of hot coconut milk. Add honey to taste. The spices in chai tea are warming in nature. Therefore, they support the spleen, and maca is nourishing and supportive to the adrenals and overall health. You can also make your own chai from the recipe in chapter 3 and add maca to it.
6:00 p.m.	Dinner is the same concept as lunch.
8:00 p.m.	Detox juice is one bunch of cilantro, one cup of coconut water, honey to taste, and the juice of half of a lemon. As an option, you can add a fresh piece of ginger or a teaspoon of Vitamineral Green from Health Force Nutritionals or chlorella. Blend ingredients.

THINGS TO AVOID

Substances which trigger immune response or inflammation must be removed from your diet until the body has healed and no longer recognizes the substances as harmful.

- **Gluten**: Stop eating gluten only if you have an autoimmune disorder, IBS, Crohon's disease, or any other inflammatory bowl disease or if you are intolerant. Otherwise eat organic gluten. This includes wheat and its varieties like spelt, kamut, farro and durum, as well as products like bulgur, and semolina. Barley, and rye also contain gluten.

  Note that **most grains are gluten-free,** when they are consumed with all of their bran, germ, and endosperm. Examples of non-gluten grains are corn, buckwheat, amaranth, quinoa, millet, Indian grass rice (montina), oats*, brown rice, sorghum, teff, and wild rice.

**Oats are gluten-free, but are frequently contaminated with wheat during growing, traveling or processing. Several companies such as Bob's Red Mill, Cream Hill Estates, GF Harvest (formerly Gluten Free Oats),* Montana Gluten Free, *and* Avena Foods *are currently among those that offer pure, uncontaminated oats.*

- ***Dairy***: Avoid all cow milk products. You may replace them with:

Dairy	Options
Milk	Coconut, almond, hazelnut, rice, hemp, or cashew milk
Butter	Coconut oil or ghee
Yogurt	Coconut or almond yogurt
Whey protein	Pea protein
Ice cream	Coconut, cashew, or almond-based ice creams
Cheese	Dairy-free cheese such as cashew, almond, and other nut-based cheeses

- ***Corn and Soy***: Regrettably, corn and soy are known allergens for some people with autoimmune and digestive disorders. Because 90 percent of corn and soy produced in the US is genetically modified it can pose health risks such as immune suppression and inflammation. Eliminate them from your diet if you feel you are sensitive to them or if you do not know if you are allergic. Otherwise, only eat organic corn and soy products.

- ***Eggs***: Eggs are a top allergen in North America, and they can be difficult to digest for many people that are sensitive or intolerant to the protein contained in eggs. Note that some people may be able to eat eggs without any issues. If you can tolerate eggs, only eat organic eggs. They are a great source of vitamin D, omega-3 fatty acids, and vitamin B.

- ***Sugar***: In addition to table sugar, avoid foods that contain sugar or high fructose corn syrup. Use stevia, honey, maple syrup, or agave as an alternative. Remove entirely from your diet artificial or modified sugars, such as Splenda, aspartame, and saccharine.

- *Caffeine*: Eliminate caffeine products as much as possible. Coffee must be removed until the gut has had an opportunity to heal and calm down. Coffee is one of the most irritating substances for the colon, it destroys the good flora in the gut, and is highly acidic. Coffee also propels the stomach to release its contents prematurely, passing food that has not been fully digested into the small intestine where it can aggravate the digestive tract. However, coffee works excellent as an enema, if you have the need to cleanse the colon or you are suffering from constipation

  If you have been using caffeine for a while, you might want to wean yourself off instead of going cold turkey. If you are gluten intolerant, use a coffee substitute such as Dande-blend or Teeccino's Dandelion Dark Roast instead of coffee. Otherwise, you may also use a coffee substitute that has gluten such as the brand Pero or other Teeccino flavors.

- *Alcohol:* While an occasional glass of wine offers a few antioxidants, excess consumption of alcohol can increase the production of C-reactive protein (CRP), a marker of inflammation. Additionally, alcohol consumption can lead to blood sugar imbalances, liver backlog, leaky gut, and overgrowth of bacteria in the small intestine. In short, the benefits of alcohol consumption do not outweigh the consequences.

- Avoid all canned, jarred, boxed, smoked, bottled, and otherwise preserved items.

- Avoid processed foods, artificial colors, and flavors. The consumption of these ingredients contributes to inflammation and toxicity of the body. As a general rule, do not consume a product if there is an ingredient on the label you cannot make at home or you aren't able to find in nature.

- Refined carbohydrates prolong the transit time of the bowel waste, resulting in above average production of putrefactive bacteria in the bowels.

- Saturated fat.
- Minimize your consumption of foods in the nightshade family of vegetables including tomatoes, white potatoes, and eggplant. Nightshades contain alkaloids that may cause gastrointestinal upset and inflammation in some people with autoimmune or digestive disorders. Stop eating them if you are sensitive to this food group or if you do not know if you are sensitive to them.

In general, this is a healthy diet plan that almost anyone can follow, even if he or she is not suffering from a chronic illness. In fact, you can follow this diet exactly as it is described above two or three times a year to do a cleanse and reset your body. Additionally, you don't need to be sick to do this program.

You may follow all the dietary guidelines listed in this book to stay healthy and prevent any disease. However, for disease prevention, you don't have to be as strict, and you will take out the extra cleansing elements from the table outlined in the "how to eat?" section of this chapter. Therefore, the diet will look something like this. (Add and remove foods and drinks to your needs.)

Time	Food
8:00 a.m. or your usual breakfast time	In a breakfast smoothie, mix one cup of mixed greens, one carrot, half an avocado (or another source of good fat such as almonds or cashews soaked overnight), one stick of celery, one cucumber, a few basil leaves, one cup coconut milk, half or one beet, half or one cup of mixed berries, and one scoop of pea protein powder. To support the spleen, try to use fresh ingredients as much as possible instead of frozen (warmer). Additionally, fresh ingredients have more life force and are more nutritious.
10:00 a.m.	Eat a snack of your choice from the foods listed in this book.
12:00 p.m.	incorporate good fats, fiber, grains (non-glutenous grains if you are gluten intolerant), legumes, vegetables, and clean animal protein, if desired. Congee can be eaten too.
3:00 p.m.	For a tea of your choice, select herbs for your tea accordingly to the effect you desire. For example, for a calming effect, you can combine chamomile, lemon balm, and catnip to support the adrenals. Select maca, adaptogen herbs, and so forth.
6:00 p.m.	For dinner, it's the same concept as lunch.

5 TIME SAVING TIPS TO HELP YOU STAY ON TRACK WITH YOUR DIET.

The following tips can help you make the transition from your current diet to the one described in this chapter:

1. *Schedule time each week to grocery shop.* If you do not schedule a time to shop, it most likely won't get done, because you will get distracted by the many competing tasks, demands, issues, and other priorities in your life.

2. *Prepare ingredients immediately.* You can get ahead on the meals from the following week by washing and chopping ingredients in bulk, slicing vegetables, cutting chicken or meat, etc. You can do this right after you arrive from the grocery store, or you can schedule a specific time to prep for the upcoming week.

3. *Cook in advance:* You can also prepare side dishes ahead of time. For example, you can cook a large batch of brown rice or beans that you can use during the week. You can also chop and place all the ingredients of your daily smoothies in individual mason jars that you can just grab when you are ready to blend. You can even prepare your meals for the next two days and heat up when you are ready to eat.

4. *Make it fun:* Food preparation does not have to be boring, you can turn your music on, listen to a podcast, lecture our audiobook, catch up on tv shows or chat with a friend on the phone while you prep.

5. *Keep snacks and simple meals handy:* celery, cucumbers, radishes, carrots, hummus, bean dip, jicama sticks, avocados, almond butter, nuts and seeds, and berries are all great snacks to keep on hand.

SAMPLE RECIPES

This book is not intended to be a compressive recipe book. However, I'm listing a few of my favorite recipes that you can use as a guideline to get you started.

BREAKFAST

Coconut Rice with Berries

Ingredients

- one cup of brown rice (soaked overnight)
- one cup of water
- one cup of coconut milk
- one teaspoon of salt
- two dates, pitted and chopped
- Fresh mix berries
- Toasted almonds

Directions:

In a medium sauce pan over high heat, combine the rice, water, coconut milk, salt, and dates. Stir until the mixture comes to a boil. Reduce the heat to simmer and cook for twenty to thirty minutes until the rice becomes tender. Serve rice and top each serving with berries and almonds.

You can replace the brown rice with quinoa, cook for fifteen minutes.

Quinoa and Berries Salad

- Half a cup of quinoa soaked overnight
- Three quarters of a cup of water
- one cup of mixed berries
- one third of a cup of almonds
- one tablespoon of maple syrup

Directions

In a small pot, add quinoa and water, bring to a boil. Cover with tight lid, reduce heat to low and simmer for fifteen minutes. Remove lid and let rest for ten minutes, fluff with a fork. Add berries, maple syrup and almonds mix well and serve.

Chocolate Quinoa Breakfast bowl

Ingredients

- one cup of uncooked white quinoa
- one cup of unsweetened almond milk
- one cup of coconut milk a pinch sea salt
- two tablespoons of unsweetened cocoa powder
- one tablespoon of maple syrup
- Optional: half a teaspoon of pure vanilla extract
- Dark chocolate chips
- Mixed berries or sliced banana

In a small pot, add quinoa and almond milk, coconut milk and a pinch of salt, bring to a boil. Cover, reduce heat to low and simmer for fifteen minutes. Remove lid and let rest for ten minutes, fluff with a fork. Add cacao powder, maple syrup, and vanilla. Stir well and serve. Top with chocolate chips, berries or bananas.

Chia Seeds and Berries Pudding

Ingredients

- two cups of almond milk
- half a cup of chia seeds

- one tablespoon of maple syrup or honey
- one teaspoon of vanilla extract
- one cup of mixed berries or cherries
- Optional: Cashews

Directions

In a mason jar or any jar with a tight lid, combine the milk, chia seeds, maple syrup, and vanilla. Shake well and set aside for fifteen minutes. Serve and top with berries and cashews.

SNACKS

White Bean Dip with Herbs

Ingredients

- A quarter of a cup of olive oil, plus additional for topping
- Three large garlic cloves diced
- one tablespoon of fresh thyme finely chopped, or one teaspoon dried
- one tablespoon of fresh rosemary finely chopped, or one teaspoon dried
- four cups of cannellini beans, soaked overnight and cooked
- two tablespoons of red wine vinegar
- Sea salt and pepper to taste
- Optional toppings: pine nuts, fresh thyme, red pepper flakes

Instructions

Add beans, olive oil, herbs, red wine vinegar and salt & pepper to a food processor. Blend on high until dip is smooth and creamy. Taste to adjust salt and pepper if needed. Pour dip into a bowl, cover, and place in the fridge for at least an hour. Remove from the fridge when ready to use and top with a drizzle of olive oil and any toppings you desire. Serve with fresh veggies, pita bread, rice crackers, or Brussel sprouts chips.

Chile-Lime Almonds Recipe

These almonds make a great topping for salads or simply as a healthy snack any day.

Ingredients

- two cups of raw almonds (soaked for a couple of hours)
- one tablespoon of olive oil
- one to two teaspoons of chili powder (depending on your taste)
- one teaspoon of salt
- one tablespoon of fresh lime juice
- one tablespoon of chopped cilantro

Add nuts and oil to a pan, sprinkle with chili powder and salt and toast for five minutes. Remove the pan from heat, add lime juice and cilantro and stir. Transfer nuts to a plate or baking sheet and let them cool. Store in airtight container.

Brussels Sprout Chips

Ingredients

- Half a pound of Brussels sprouts, thinly sliced
- one tablespoon of olive oil
- one teaspoon of garlic powder
- sea salt
- Ground black pepper
- Roasted Garlic Hummus or white bean dip, for dipping

Directions

Preheat oven to 400°. In a large bowl, toss Brussels sprouts with olive oil, and garlic powder. Season with salt and pepper. Spread in an even layer on a medium baking sheet. Bake ten minutes, toss, and bake eight to ten minutes more, until crisp and golden. Serve with Roasted Garlic Hummus or white bean dip for dipping.

Roasted Garlic Hummus

Ingredients

- four cups of chickpeas (soaked overnight and strained)
- one tablespoon of lemon juice
- half a cup of tahini
- one teaspoon of cumin
- one and half teaspoons of sea salt, plus more for roasted garlic
- half a teaspoon of red pepper flakes
- Freshly ground black pepper

- Three quarter cup of olive oil, plus more for topping and roasted garlic
- Paprika, for garnish
- Freshly chopped parsley, for garnish
- one head of garlic

Directions

Preheat oven to 400°. Place in a large pot cover with water by at least an inch. Bring to a boil then cover and reduce heat. Let simmer until tender and falling apart, about one hour. If using, roast garlic: Cut the top off the head of garlic. Drizzle with olive oil and season with salt and pepper. Wrap in foil and place in a shallow dish. Roast until golden and soft, about forty minutes. Let cool then remove garlic cloves. Drain chickpeas and place in the bowl of a food processor. Add garlic, lemon juice, tahini, cumin, salt, red pepper flakes, and pepper. Blend until smooth. With the food processor running, slowly add in olive oil until hummus is at desired consistency. Plate hummus in a bowl and top with olive oil, paprika, and parsley.

Spicy Roasted Chickpeas

Ingredients

- two cups cooked of chickpeas (soaked overnight before cooking)
- one and a half teaspoons of olive oil
- a quarter of a teaspoon of salt
- a quarter of teaspoon of black pepper
- three forth of a teaspoon of chili powder
- a quarter of a teaspoon paprika
- a quarter of a teaspoon garlic powder
- a dash of cayenne pepper

Directions

Preheat oven to 425 degrees F. Pat the chickpeas dry between two paper towels and be sure to remove any loose skins. Pour the chickpeas on a baking sheet lined with parchment paper and mist with olive oil. Use your hands or a spoon to toss the chickpeas. In a small bowl, combine the spices and combine well. Sprinkle the mixture onto the chickpeas and toss to coat. Bake for twenty-five minutes, stirring the chickpeas after fifteen minutes.

Other quick and easy snacks:

- Apple slices with almond butter
- Avocado and salsa with toast
- Banana and almond butter sandwich
- Dried seaweed
- Non-dairy yogurt with berries

DRINKS / SMOOTHIES

The following drinks can be consumed throughout the day instead of soft-drinks and other high sugar drinks.

Anti-inflammatory Ginger Tea

Juice one or more pieces of ginger, in total about the size of a carrot. Combine about a quarter of a cup of ginger juice with twelve ounces of hot water, one tablespoon of honey, the juice of a quarter of a lemon or lime (squeeze the juice into the cup and then drop the rind), and a pinch of cayenne (less if you are unable to tolerate the heat).

If you do not own a juicer, use the infusion method below. Or buy organic fresh-squeezed ginger juice (not from concentrate). Make sure it has not been diluted with water or other juices. I have found the "Ginger People" brand to be effective.

Infusion method: Grate or chop a ginger root about the size of your thumb as finely you can. Steep in eight to twelve ounces of hot water for two to three hours, covered with tight lid to preserve the essential oils.

Hibiscus Lavender Lemonade Recipe

Ingredients

- three cups of water
- one and half cups lemon juice
- Honey or maple syrup to taste
- two tablespoons dried lavender flowers
- one and a half teaspoons of dried hibiscus petals

Directions

Mix three cups of water and lemon juice in a large pitcher. Refrigerate until chilled. Bring remaining three cups water, sugar, lavender, and hibiscus petals to a boil in a saucepan. Reduce heat to medium-low and simmer for ten minutes. Remove from heat and allow to cool. Strain lavender and hibiscus from liquid and pour into a pitcher with lemon water. Add sweetener to taste (not too much). Refrigerate until cold.

Carrot, Apple and Celery Smoothie

- one apple, cut in quarters away from the core
- one carrot, cut in half
- one stalk of celery, cut in half
- Juice of one lemon
- one small piece of fresh ginger root
- one cup of coconut water

Directions

Place ingredients in your high-speed blender. Blend on high for one to two minutes, stopping intermittently if ingredients need to be mixed.

Pear and Ginger Anti-inflammatory and Digestion Aid Smoothie

Ingredients

- one pear or apple cored
- half of a fennel bulb
- one slice of fresh ginger
- one cup of packed power greens like kale, chard and spinach
- Half a cucumber with peel (unless is not organic)
- Half a cup of water

Directions:

Place all ingredients in high-speed blender and blend until smooth.

Cherry Smoothie

Ingredients

- one cup of frozen or fresh pitted cherries
- a quarter of a cup of raspberries
- three quarters of a cup of coconut water
- Optional: one teaspoon of chia seeds
- Optional: one teaspoon of hemp seeds
- Half a teaspoon of vanilla extract

Directions:

Place all ingredients in high-speed blender and blend until smooth.

Power Greens and Apple Smoothie

Ingredients

- one green apple cored and quartered
- half a cup of coconut water
- one cup of packed power greens like kale, chard, and spinach
- a quarter of a lemon seeded (or more, to taste)
- half a cucumber
- Optional: one teaspoon of honey or maple syrup

Directions:

Place all ingredients in high-speed blender and blend until smooth.

Green Chai Smoothie

Ingredients

- one banana
- Half a teaspoon of ground ginger
- A quarter of a teaspoon ground cinnamon
- A quarter of a teaspoon ground cardamom
- An eight of a teaspoon ground nutmeg
- one tablespoon of natural almond butter
- two cups of packed power greens like kale, chard and spinach
- one cup of unsweetened almond milk
- Optional: half a teaspoon of vanilla extract

Directions:

Place all ingredients in high-speed blender and blend until smooth.

Tomato Juice

Ingredients:

- One or two tomatoes
- one celery stick
- half a cucumber
- one radish
- one small bunch of cilantro
- one carrot
- juice of half a lemon
- a pinch of salt

Directions:

Place all ingredients in high-speed blender and blend until smooth.

LUNCH / DINNER

Lentil Immune and Antimicrobial Soup

This soup contains thyme, garlic and cayenne, all antimicrobial herbs and the spices. It is also a rich source of antioxidants and nutrients that support digestion and immunity and combat inflammation (it is wonderful substitute for chicken soup for those that are vegetarian or vegan).

Ingredients

- eight cups of vegetable stock or water

- one tablespoon of avocado oil (or coconut oil)
- one onion, diced
- four to eight cloves garlic, minced
- one cup of sliced carrots
- one slice of astragalus root
- one cup of shiitake mushrooms, sliced
- one cup of chopped celery
- one tablespoon of dried thyme
- a quarter to half a teaspoon of cayenne pepper
- two bay leaves
- half a cup of quinoa, brown rice or another gluten-free grain (soaked overnight)
- half of a cup of green lentils

Directions

Bring the vegetable broth or water to a boil in a large pot. Meanwhile, heat the avocado oil in a skillet and add the onion, garlic, and vegetables. Sauté over low heat until soft and aromatic. Add contents of skillet to broth along with astragalus root, shiitake mushrooms, and herbs. Add grain and lentils. Simmer, covered, for an hour. Remove astragalus before serving.

Super Immune Boosting Brown Rice and Astragalus Soup

Ingredients

- Three quarters of a cup brown rice, washed and soaked overnight
- eight cups of water or stock of your choice
- one ounce of astragalus root
- one 1 ½ inch piece of ginger, peeled and julienned
- three or four dried shiitake mushrooms, cut into thin slices with scissors (no stems)
- sesame oil (preferably), or other similar oil
- one small onion, peeled and diced
- one cup of daikon radish, diced
- one cup of carrots, diced
- salt, tamari sauce, white miso to taste
- two green onions, slivered, as garnish

Directions

Bring the water or stock to a boil in a soup pot. Add a pinch of salt, the rice, astragalus root, ginger, and shiitake mushrooms. Bring back to a boil, then reduce to a low simmer and simmer about one hour and twenty minutes, or until the rice is partly dissolved into a creamy broth. Add more water as needed to make the soup the consistency you prefer. While the rice is simmering, heat a sauté pan and sauté the vegetables with a pinch of salt for about five minutes, or until they begin to be soft. Add the vegetables to the rice pot, stir and simmer about five minutes more. Taste and season, adding a tablespoon of white miso if you like, or a little bit of tamari sauce. Remove the astragalus root from the rice.

Garnish with green onions, pickled vegetables, or other toppings that appeal to you. Tastes excellent reheated the next day! To make things easier, you can cook in a crock pot instead of stove top.

Roasted Broccoli with Sage

Ingredients:

- one pound of broccoli florets
- half a red onion, sliced
- eight fresh sage leaves torn (one teaspoon dried)
- two tablespoons extra-virgin olive oil
- half a teaspoon of salt
- half teaspoon of garlic salt
- a quarter of a teaspoon ground black pepper
- Optional: a quarter of a cup pine or pistachio nuts.

Directions:

Preheat oven to 400 degrees F. Spread broccoli in a single layer on a baking sheet. Sprinkle onion and sage leaves over broccoli; drizzle with olive oil. Sprinkle salt, garlic salt, and black pepper over broccoli mixture; toss to coat. Roast in the preheated oven until broccoli is browned and crisp, twenty to thirty minutes.

Spicy Burdock Root & Carrot Stir-Fry

Ingredients

- one large burdock root
- one carrot
- half to one whole dried red chili, seeds removed

- one tablespoon of honey, maple syrup or agave
- one tablespoon of white wine vinegar
- one and a half tablespoons Tamari sauce
- half a tablespoon sesame seeds (optional)

Directions:

Scrub the burdock root, cut into matchsticks and soak in water. Rinse until water runs clear. Cut carrots into matchsticks as well. Measure out the sweetener, vinegar and soy sauce. Heat sesame oil in a pan and sauté burdock, carrot and red chili on medium heat until carrot is soft. The burdock root will remain a bit harder. Add in sweetener and vinegar first. Mix well for a minute or two, then add in tamari sauce. Stir fry until tamari sauce begins to caramelize and gives off a nice smell. Stop the heat and sprinkle on sesame seeds. Goes well with brown rice and leftovers can be used for lunches.

Healthy Pumpkin Soup Recipe

To help you stay healthy during the fall and winter days, incorporate pumpkin soup (and pumpkin in general) in your diet. Pumpkin is an extremely nutrient-dense food; meaning it is full of vitamins and minerals. Also, the spices in pumpkin soup are antimicrobial. However, do not limit yourself to pumpkin soup, as there are many creative ways pumpkin can be incorporated into your diet, including desserts, soups, salads, and preserves.

Ingredients

- One an a half tablespoons extra-virgin olive oil (or coconut oil)
- one cup of chopped onion
- three garlic cloves minced
- three cups of (packed) pumpkin
- two cups of low-salt vegetable broth

- two teaspoons of honey, maple syrup or agave
- half a teaspoon of ground allspice
- half a teaspoon of dried crushed red pepper
- one and a half cups of unsweetened coconut milk
- Salt and pepper
- Pumpkin seeds (for garnish)

Directions:

Heat the oil in a heavy large pot over medium heat. Add the onion and garlic. Sauté until golden (about ten minutes). Add the pumpkin, broth, sweetener, allspice, and crushed red pepper. Bring to a boil. Reduce the heat. Cover and simmer until flavors blend (about thirty minutes). Working in batches, puree the soup in a blender until smooth. Return the soup to the pot. Bring the soup to a simmer, thinning with coconut milk to the desired consistency. Season to taste with salt and pepper. Ladle the soup into bowls. Sprinkle with the pumpkin seeds, drizzle with a teaspoon of coconut milk and serve.

CHAPTER TEN

Restore Gut and Immune Health

A path to health is paved with good intestines.
—S. A. ROGERS

It is said that If you want to fix your health, start with your gut. The human gut is an ecosystem consisting of a significant number of bacteria living in harmony with the host. Several studies confirm that gut microbiota (good bacteria) is engaged in dynamic interaction with the immune system. Furthermore, evidence indicates that intestinal microflora has protective, metabolic, trophic, and immunological functions. In fact, 20 percent of thyroid gland function depends on this friendly flora. When one or more steps in this fine interaction fail, autoimmune or auto-inflammatory diseases may occur. Therefore, improving the health of your gut flora will strengthen your immune function, consequently helping you fight and prevent diseases.

Now that you know how important the gut is for immunity, what can you do about it? To start with, feed your gut bacteria the right food and learn how to fertilize your healthy inner garden. Give them whole, fresh, real foods; fermented foods and drinks like kombucha and kefir (only if you do not have candida); and a good probiotic supplement that contains fructooligosaccharides (FOS). FOS is a fiber that feeds and helps good bacteria thrive. It is found naturally in many fruits, grains, and vegetables. FOS has also been shown to increase absorption of minerals such as calcium, help you feel full, reduce the risk of colon cancer and, keep you regular.

Additionally, to keep your gut healthy minimize the following:

- A junk food diet: A nutrient-poor diet promotes the growth of the wrong (bad) bacteria and yeast in the gut, leading to a damaged ecosystem.
- Medication overuse: Anti-inflammatories, antibiotics, acid-blocking drugs, and steroids damage the intestine and block normal digestive function.
- Infections and gut imbalances: These include small intestinal bacterial overgrowth, yeast overgrowth, and parasites.
- Toxic overload: This includes mercury and mold toxins.
- Inadequate digestive enzymes: Stress, acid-blocking medications, and zinc deficiencies can all contribute to lack of adequate digestive enzyme function.
- *Eating too many raw foods.* Digesting raw vegetables takes a lot of energy, and if you are already having digestive issues, too many raw vegetables can exaggerate the problem.
- Stress: Chronic stress (including depression and anxiety) alters your gut nervous system, creating a leaky gut and changing its normal bacteria. Particularly, eating while under stress can harm your gut.

Additionally, people with autoimmune disorders, allergies, and some chronic illnesses often have a what is called a leaky gut, or "intestinal permeability." As discussed in chapter 6, this condition is caused by toxins and infections in which the lining of the small intestine becomes unhealthy and may have cracks or holes, causing undigested food particles, toxic waste products, and bacteria to "leak" through the intestines and go into the bloodstream. Therefore, it is imperative to restore the lining of the intestines to be able to regain health. Fortunately, some herbs can help us do this.

HERBS TO RESTORE THE LINING OF THE INTESTINES

A few of the best-known herbs to restore the lining of the intestine are:

- *Marshmallow* has been used for centuries to treat many illnesses, such as coughs and colds, infections, and to improve digestion. Research suggests that marshmallow is effective to treat digestive disorders, including leaky gut syndrome by restoring the integrity of the gut lining by forming a protective layer around small junctions. Also it seems to be beneficial for people suffering from other forms of inflammatory bowel diseases, including ulcerative colitis and Crohn's disease. Additionally, marshmallow has been shown to help lower or prevent heartburn, stomach ulcer symptoms, diarrhea, and constipation. Reason being, marshmallow coats the inside of the stomach and prevents acid from causing discomfort and "burning."

- *Slippery elm* has been used successfully for many years to treat wounds, burns, boils, psoriasis, and other external skin conditions. Similarly, to marshmallow, studies have shown that slippery elm also helps protect against ulcers and excess acidity. Additionally, it has been shown to improve constipation, bloating, diarrhea, and other issues associated with IBS and diverticulitis. Slippery elm is an endangered species. Therefore, use with caution or use marshmallow root instead.

- *Licorice* is anti-inflammatory and has many antioxidants. It is also an adaptogen, and it has been used for thousands of years for many uses, including for coughs, adrenal fatigue, leaky gut, and heartburn.

- Many of *plantain's* active constituents have shown antibacterial and antimicrobial properties as well as being anti-inflammatory and antitoxic. It has been used for hundreds of years to relieve the discomfort of bee stings and insect bites, stop the itching of poison ivy and other allergic rashes, and promote healing in sores and bruises.

- *Chamomile* is considered to be one of the most ancient and versatile medicinal herbs known to humanity. So much so that it is often referred to as a panacea. Chamomile is commonly used for liver cleanse, heals digestive issues, and improves many different health conditions, including anxiety and depression, allergies or hay fever, muscle spasms, PMS and other menstrual disorders, insomnia, skin disorders, ulcers, wounds, gastrointestinal disorders, arthritis, rheumatic, pain, and hemorrhoids, amongst many others. It is also an anti-inflammatory.

- *Peppermint* provides a cooling sensation and has a calming effect on the body. It also contains antimicrobial properties, can help freshen bad breath, and soothe nausea, headaches, and digestive issues. It also has a soothing effect on the gastric lining and colon because of its ability to reduce muscle spasms. In fact, it has been shown to treat IBS effectively.

Select a few of these herbs and create an herbal tea formula. Make sure your formula contains one demulcent herb such as marshmallow, slippery elm, or licorice. Or you can use the digestive formula that I have designed specifically for this program. You can find it on my website at https://www.moongazingapothecary.com/autoimmune-herbal-supplements Your other option is to buy the individual herbs to create your formula or buy a preformulated digestive herbal tea from a reliable source.

Drink two cups of this tea every day. Make with one-half ounce of herb for sixteen ounces of water. Simmer on low heat for twenty minutes (covered). Dose and consistency are critical for this tea to work. (You will need to take this tea for at least three months.)

Always buy organic and from a reliable company such as Herb-Pharm, Gaia Herbs, or my brand, Moongazing Herbal Apothecary. Remember, the quality of the herb is directly correlated to its effectiveness.

Also, one of the leading causes of intestinal permeability is imbalanced flora in your gut, including an overgrowth of yeast and candida. Therefore, another critical step in the process of restoring your gut health will be improving your gut flora. Thus, it is essential to add to this regimen a good *soil-based* probiotic supplement (dose of at least 15 billion per day) and antimicrobial herbs such as barberry, oregano, goldenseal, or Oregon grape root. When choosing a probiotic, select one that contains spore-forming bacteria. This type of probiotic is able to bypass your small intestine and colonize your colon and large intestine.

MORE ON IMMUNE HEALTH

Normal functioning of the immune system is critical to our health. Therefore, immune function should always be at the top of your list of health priorities. The immune system doesn't just keep colds and flu away. It is also the body's best defense against any disease. Your daily habits—including the foods you eat, exercise and sleep routines, environmental toxins, and emotional stress—have a significant effect on your immune function and can conspire to weaken immunity. To support your immune system, try to follow these lifestyle suggestions:

- Don't smoke.
- Eat a diet high in whole grains, vegetables, fruits, and good fats and low in saturated fat, such as the one described in chapter 3.
- Reduce or eliminate refined sugar intake. Eating or drinking too much sugar suppresses immune system cells that attack bacteria. Instead moderately use sugar substitutes such as honey, agave, and maple syrup.
- Exercise regularly but not in excess. Studies show that at least thirty minutes of exercise on most days of the week increases immune function. However, excessive exercise regimes can temporarily hinder immune function.
- Maintain a healthy weight.
- Manage your blood pressure.

- If you drink alcohol, drink only in moderation.
- Get adequate sleep.
- Reduce or eliminate your coffee intake (one or two cups per day). Caffeine may raise levels of the stress hormone cortisol, which suppresses the immune system. If you're a coffee drinker, try substituting green tea for coffee. Green tea has less than half as much caffeine as coffee and is rich in antioxidants. There are also quite a few coffee substitute products that may be used as safe alternatives to coffee. Teeccino or Dandy Blend are great herbal substitutes.

Likewise, quite a few herbs support and restore the immune system, including adaptogens, which are substances that help the body better cope with mental, environmental, and physical stress. There is much evidence that immune support herbs act to stimulate or modulate the immune system. Immune modulators bring about increased resistance through a nonspecific self-regulating process. These herbs work to increase innate immunity and provide vital support to the immune system. On the other hand, immune stimulants boost the activity of the immune system but are not known to normalize excessive immune response. Consequently, they are not recommended for people who have autoimmune disorders. Instead people with autoimmune diseases should only use immune-modulating herbs.

The following list covers some of the best-researched immune and adaptogen herbs.

HERB	HEALTH BENEFITS	Type
Astragalus	Astragalus root is one of the most potent immune-boosting plants. It is a Chinese herb that's been used for centuries to strengthen the body's internal systems, and it specifically helps with colds and upper respiratory infections. Its greatest strength is preventing and protecting cells against cell death and other harmful elements, such as free radicals and oxidation. Do not take astragalus while you have a fever.	Stimulant (adaptogen)

HERB	HEALTH BENEFITS	Type
Ashwagandha	This herb is popular in Aryuvedic medicine, and it has been used for more than 2,500 years. It has many health benefits, including thyroid modulating and neuroprotective. It strengthens the immune system, enhances stamina and endurance, improves fertility and sexual function, relieves adrenal fatigue, balances blood sugar levels, and improves cognitive function. It relieves stress and lowers cortisol levels. It is anti-anxiety, antidepressant, and anti-inflammatory.	Modulates (adaptogen)
Black Elderberry	Elderberry (Sambucus) is used for its antioxidant activity to lower cholesterol, improve vision, boost the immune system, improve heart health, and treat tonsillitis and respiratory, bacterial, and viral infections. Also evidence suggests that chemicals in elderflower and berries may help reduce swelling in mucous membranes, including the sinuses, and help relieve nasal congestion. Elderberry may have anti-inflammatory, antiviral, anti-influenza, and anticancer properties. A study found that using a standardized elderberry extract could shorten the duration of flu by about three days. Another study found that a lozenge with elderberry extract helped reduce flu symptoms when taken within twenty-four hours of symptoms starting. In the lab, one study suggested that elderberry could kill the H1N1 virus ("swine flu") in test tubes.	Stimulant

HERB	HEALTH BENEFITS	Type
Echinancea	Echinacea stimulates the immune system and prevents and treats upper respiratory tract infections. Studies suggest that it stimulates cells in the body whose primary function is to fight invading particles and organisms. White blood cells and spleen cells increase in number when echinacea is taken. North American Indians and early settlers used echinacea as an antimicrobial for relief of infections and pain and for reducing symptoms of snakebites. Others have used echinacea for relief of scarlet fever, syphilis, malaria, blood poisoning, and diphtheria.	Stimulant
Eluthero	In Chinese medicine, eluthero (also known as Siberian ginseng) is used to prevent respiratory tract infections, colds, and flu and to increase energy, longevity, and vitality. Double-blind studies have found that a specific product containing eluthero reduced the severity and length of colds when taken within seventy-two hours of symptoms starting. Another study found that healthy people who took eluthero for four weeks had an increase of T-cells, which may indicate a strengthening of their immune systems. It is widely used in Russia as an adaptogen.	Modulates (adaptogen)

HERB	HEALTH BENEFITS	Type
Ginseng (Panax)	Canadian researchers found that ginseng, an herb widely used in Chinese medicine, is proving successful in reducing the number and severity of colds in research subjects. Ginseng also improves stamina and stress resistance and enhances the ability to endure physical strain, resist disease, and perform tests of mental sharpness. It is also an anti-inflammatory. It boosts metabolism; helps with depression, anxiety, and chronic fatigue, and erectile dysfunction; lowers blood sugar; relieves menopause symptoms; improves lung function; and prevents cancer.	Modulates (adaptogen)
Green Tea	Green tea is of great scientific interest due to its potentially positive effects on the mind and body. For example, there is evidence that it can help strengthen the immune system. By enhancing immune agents, protecting against oxidative stress that can damage cells, and preventing autoimmune disorders like rheumatoid arthritis, green tea is thought to be highly beneficial.	Modulates

HERB	HEALTH BENEFITS	Type
Holy Basil	Also known as tulsi, it's used as a remedy for anxiety, adrenal fatigue, hypothyroidism, unbalanced blood sugar, and acne. Scientists have proven that it helps protect organs and tissues against chemical stress from industrial pollutants and heavy metals and physical stress from prolonged physical exertion and ischemia. It is an antibacterial, antiviral, carminative, diuretic, expectorant, antidepressant, antioxidant, and galactagogue (promotes mother's milk). Additionally it has been shown that helps fight cancer, balances hormones, and relieves congestion and other symptoms of respiratory conditions.	Modulates (adaptogen)
Licorice	It is antiviral, antidiuretic, antihistamine, anti-inflammatory, antioxidant, antitumor, demulcent, expectorant, and hepaprotective.	Modulate (adaptogen)
Maca	Antioxidant-rich, it increases strength, energy, stamina, cognitive function such as memory and mood, and libido and sexual function. It balances estrogen levels and boosts male fertility.	(adaptogen)
Rhodiola	Also known as rose root, it is antidepressant, antioxidant, antiviral, nervine, mild central nervous system stimulant, antiarrythmic (protects against irregular heartbeats), cardioprotective, and neuroprotective.	Stimulant (adaptogen)
Rose hips	Rose hips contain 50 percent more vitamin C than oranges. Because of their high vitamin C content, they are an excellent immune system booster and can help prevent infections from both bacteria and viruses. They are often used as a supplement to prevent or treat a cold.	Stimulant

HERB	HEALTH BENEFITS	Type
Shiitake Mushroom	Some of the most potent immunosupportive agents come from mushrooms. There are mushrooms that kill viruses, bacteria, yeast, and even ones that kill cancer. A new study from the University of Florida showed increased immunity in people who ate a cooked shiitake mushroom every day for four weeks.	Modulates
Reishi Mushroom	Nicknamed "the Great Protector," red reishi mushroom has been used for centuries for its numerous health benefits. Proven to be a powerful immune modulator, this mushroom has been shown to contain health-giving compounds that regulate antibody production, protecting you against cold and flu viruses. It can also be taken during a cold or flu to help speed up recovery and minimize a virus' effect. It works best when taken regularly to prevent viruses from taking hold in the first place. Make sure to choose a product rich in polysaccharides, sterols, and other compounds that support the immune system.	Modulates (adaptogen)

Overall your first line of defense against disease is a healthy lifestyle. Nevertheless, if you are in need of additional immune support, the previously mentioned herbs are your best bet to help restore your immune function. Immune support herbs are best when taken regularly to prevent illness. However, it is helpful to take a one-week break from herbal immune stimulants after taking them for about one month and then begin taking them again.

CHAPTER ELEVEN

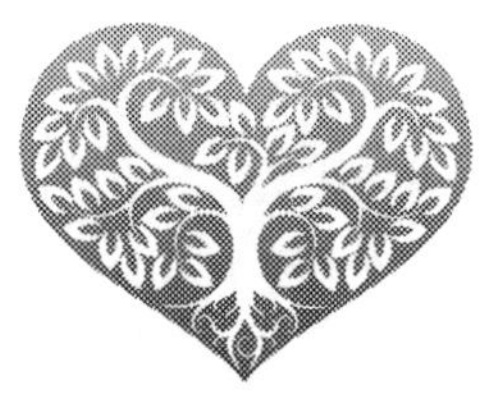

Minimize Environmental Toxins

There is only one healing power, and this is nature.
—ARTHUR SCHOPENHAUER

As discussed in detail in chapters 5 and 6, many everyday environmental factors such as toxins and endocrine disruptors have been linked to the increase in the last few decades of asthma, allergies, autoimmune disorders, and chronic illness. That is why it is important that you create an environment that supports our health.

Start with identifying and making a list of all chemical and metals you are being exposed to and eliminate them as much as possible. Here are some suggestions:

- Purchase organic or wildcrafted produce. In particular, replace in your diet conventionally grown strawberries, apples, celery, cucumbers, corn, soy, grapes, spinach, and potatoes since they contain the highest amounts of pesticides.

- Replace Teflon, stainless steel, and plastic cooking utensils with less toxic options, such as glass dishes, ceramic-coated pots and pans, and cast-iron skillets.
- Use wood utensils to cook instead of plastic-coated or metal utensils.
- Use chlorine-free parchment paper instead of aluminum foil.
- Replace your plastic food storage containers with glass containers. If you use plastic, use BPA-free plastic (including storage bags).
- Remove chemicals such as fluoride and chlorine from your water.
- Add air-cleaning houseplants to your home such as aloe vera, spider plant, dracaena, ficus, peace lily, Boston fern, snake plant, and bamboo palm, or use an air purifier.
- Minimize your use of conventional personal care items such as shampoos, lotions, cleansers, makeup, antiperspirants, and perfumes and replace them with clean brands.
- Use EMF protection devices.

THE HEALING POWER OF NATURE

Moreover, you can utilize nature to counteract the effects of environmental toxins and heal and prevent chronic illness and autoimmune disorders. A growing body of research is now demonstrating that exposure to nature or its elements can result in beneficial effects, including but not limited to improved cognition and psychological well-being, lowered blood pressure, reduced stress, and faster healing. In fact, a simple view of nature out of a window can help patients heal faster. For example, in one study, patients recovering from gallbladder surgery that had a view of trees outside their windows recovered more quickly than patients whose windows faced a brick wall.[84]

Furthermore, research shows that nature also has a positive effect on your immune system. "Your immune system doesn't only communicate with other organs and systems in your body; it also communicates with the outside world. It is a sensory organ that is made to receive information that you are not able to consciously receive," states Clemens G. Arvay in his book, *The Biophilia Effect.*[7]

He goes on and states, "One day spent in the wilderness increases the number of our natural killer cells in the blood by 40 percent on average. If you spend two days in a row in a wooded area, you can raise the number of your natural killer cells by more than 50 percent." What is more impressive is that research shows that those who spent just one day in the forest will have more natural killer cells in their bodies for seven days after, even if they did not go back during that time. Other studies on the effects of nature on our well-being have shown:

- Walking in the forest decreases blood glucose levels of type 2 diabetics. Moreover, merely being present in the forest lowers blood sugar.[85]
- Nature alleviates pain, even if only observed by a window.[84] In fact, significant reduction of a pain was observed even if the images of nature are transmitted via movies, pictures, or sound recordings.
- A simple view of trees in hospitals reduces postoperative complications.[84]
- The presence of a houseplant can improve recovery after surgery and reduce the need of painkillers.[84]
- Sunlight enhances the release of serotonin, "the happy hormone." Serotonin is known to promote feelings of peace, serenity, and satisfaction. It also eliminates anxiety, aggression, and excessive worry.
- In senior citizen and geriatric homes, residents who regularly spent time in gardens need less painkillers and antidepressants.
- Walking in the forest drastically lowers stress hormone levels.[86]
- Regularly spending time in nature protects against sleep problems.[86]

- Nature supports heart health. Scientists in Japan and Korea demonstrated that walking in the woods as well as passively observing nature reduces blood pressure and calms the heartbeat.[86]
- DHEA, a hormone produced in the adrenals, is enhanced when spending time in nature. This hormone is considered a "heart protector" substance as well as a precursor to both male and female sex hormones.

Additionally, a technique named *earthing*, also known as *grounding*, can promote health. It is based on scientific research that demonstrated that connecting to earth's electrical energy supports physical well-being. In particular, it has an impressive positive effect on inflammation.

Additionally, in 2004 the *Journal of Alternative and Complementary Medicine* reported, "Earthing during sleep resynchronizes cortisol secretion more in alignment with its natural, normal rhythm." Other studies also reported numerous positive results, including the following amongst others: improved sleep, decreased pain and inflammation, reduced feelings of stress, and improvements in gastrointestinal symptoms.

Earthing can be very simple and affordable, and it can be achieved in many ways: standing, sitting, lying, or walking with direct skin contact with the ground. It is as simple as finding a piece of earth or going to the beach, kicking off your shoes, and spending twenty to thirty minutes in contact with the earth. There are also earthing products such as shoes and bedsheets as a convenient alternative to maintain contact with the earth during work, rest, or sleep.

Finally, work on bringing balance to all your nine environments discussed in chapter 5, in particular, the relationship environment. Just as some people help you to reach your full potential, negative people can drag you down with them and impact your health. Whether it is in the form of negativity, cruelty, or the victim syndrome, toxic people create stress and strife that needs to be evaded as much as possible. Equality essential to your health is the memetic environment and minimizing your exposure to the negative emotional content of the news, films, books, and television shows are critical.

According to Jack Canfield, best-selling author and co-creator of *Chicken Soup for the Soul* books, there are three things you can do to transform an environment:[87]

- Add something such as a new friend or new equipment, for example, computer, phone, desk, belief, habit, and so on.
- Delete something, including but not limited to a negative person, a limiting belief, clutter, a bad habit, sugar, and so forth.
- Modify something, like painting a room, setting a boundary with a friend or family member, going to different places to eat out, and so on.

As with the environmental toxins, review each of the nine environments. (The list is in chapter 6.) Identify and make a list of all the changes you could make in each one that would enhance the quality of your life, and slowly start incorporating these changes in your life.

Remember, when working on restoring health, it is very important to make changes to your environment too. Otherwise, if you keep your environment the same while you are trying to change, you will create blockages, and it will slow down or stop your progress. I know it sounds like a lot of changes, but there's no need to stress or get overwhelmed. In part three of this book, I will walk you through a step-by-step process to make all these changes.

CHAPTER TWELVE

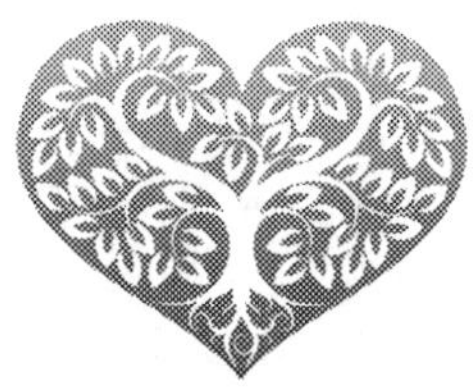

Improve Your Emotional Health

The individual who no longer has a rigid mind has found freedom. Life can be so easy. Refuse to let go, and you are a person drowning; the more you struggle, the faster you sink.

—GEORGE OHSAWA

An essential step toward healing your body is to learn how to manage stress and other negative emotions. In fact, a course in miracles states, "All disease comes from a state of non-forgiveness"[88] and it is often said that pain is the manifestation of fear in the body and the withholding of love from ourselves and others. On the other hand, joy and ecstasy reflect an outpouring of love for ourselves and everything else in the universe.

Besides, we are always only dealing with our perceptions. Scientific evidence describes that our emotions shape our reality at a molecular level and every thought we think is creating our future. Consequently, this may have several effects on the condition of our health and the overall life we experience.[89] In particular, resentment, anger, criticism, depression, guilt, and other negative emotions have a damaging effect on our health and also will attract more negative situations into our lives. This is because what you regularly think becomes your reality.

Therefore, unplesant thoughts (low vibration) show up as disease, unfortunate events, and other negativity in your life. The only path to health and a good life is to create peace and harmony in our lives. Peace and harmony come from high-vibration emotions such as appreciation, joy, and excitement. The higher we vibrate, the more joy we feel. Furthermore, by holding these types of emotions, you attract similar high-vibration (positive) experiences in your life and can create any experience you wish. You can be in this constant state of bliss. It is as simple as being willing to:

- Take 100 percent responsibility for your life. No more blaming or complaining about anything.
- Let go of the past, all resentments, and bitterness.
- Forgive yourself and others. (For exercises to help you forgive, see Appendix D and E).
- Be willing to live in the present moment as much as possible.
- Live with constant gratitude and appreciation of what is.
- Loving your self.

The good news is that there are many techniques that can help you manage negative emotions or uplift you. For example, researchers have found that the simple process of journal writing about stressful incidents improves immune function. There are hundreds of other different techniques to manage stress and improve your mood, including yoga, guided imagery, qigong, and meditation.

Likewise, there are many ways to maintain good emotional health and let go of past hurts and limiting beliefs such as emotional freedom technique (EFT), the Sedona method, the work from Byron Katie, dialectical behavioral therapy (DBT), cognitive behavioral therapy (CBT), compassion focus therapy (CFT), Gestalt therapy, neurolinguistic programming (NLP), and many more. To improve your health, find one or more techniques that work best for you and try to work on improving your emotional health daily.

More importantly, you can do a few simple things on a daily basis to ensure that you are continually experiencing high vibrational emotions and experiences:

- Release negative emotions as they come up, whether through a conversation with a friend, writing, drawing, or some form of artistic expression. Process them and let them go. The longer you ruminate on negative thoughts, the more you will see them manifest in your reality and your health. I have found the total truth process and the feeling exercise outlined in appendix D and E are great tools to help you process negative emotions and to release resentment.

- Practice mindfulness meditation on a regular basis. (Daily is better.) Not only does meditation help you be in the present moment, it also dispels negative thinking and rewires your brain for positive thoughts. Remember, every thought you think and anything you say throughout the day is an affirmation. Therefore, it is essential to be mindful of our thoughts all day long.

- Surround yourself with positive people. Emotions are contagious. Allowing negative people into your life will only bring you and your energy vibrations down and can also hurt your spirit. Therefore, keep the company of those who inspire, uplift, and encourage you to live the best life possible.

- Find ways to gain spiritual awareness and connection to the divine, such as meditation, mindfulness, stillness, creativity, walking in the park or beach, and so on.

- Find joy in the present moment. Being happy doesn't mean that everything is perfect. It means you've decided to look beyond the imperfections. Enjoy the little things, such as your well-being, your pets, listening to the rain, and so on. Moreover, the only way to create a new healthy future is to focus on and appreciate the present moment.

- Develop an attitude of gratitude. Make a habit of expressing gratitude and appreciation in all parts of your life on a daily basis. Be grateful for both the big and small things alike. I have found that thinking why I'm thankful for a particular object, person, or situation, makes me feel gratitude even more deeply.

- Through meditation, send peace and love to the world (love and kindness meditation). Good feelings toward others release oxytocin, endorphins, and other biochemicals in the brain that generate feelings of warmth and euphoria. It also contributes to the improvement of the planet. Volunteer work also promotes these feelings.

- Find your purpose and live it. When you feel as if your life has meaning, research shows that you may be less likely to develop sleep problems, have a heart attack, or die prematurely.[90] I found Jack Canfield's works (books, seminar, courses, and so forth) to be instrumental in helping you find your life purpose and achieve the life of your dreams.

- Use process affirmations and visualization daily. Affirm positive beliefs about yourself and the life you would like to experience and visualize and feel what this life looks like. If you would like to learn more about this technique, I recommend reading Jack Canfield's book, *Key to Living the Law of Attraction*.

- Be mindful of what you watch on TV and the music you listen to. The news, negative shows and movies, and negative song lyrics generate low vibrations that may contribute to experiencing overwhelming feelings, sadness, clutter, addictions, control, anger, and so on.

- Make time to read a positive book or article each day, even if is only for twenty minutes.

- Dedicate an hour a day to do an activity that brings you joy. It could be painting, writing, playing music, dancing, and so forth.

- Dedicate an hour a day to personal development. This is also very useful. You can divide this hour like twenty minutes of exercise, twenty minutes of reading, ten minutes of gratitude, and ten minutes of meditation.

- First thing in the morning, listen to one or more of the songs listed below (all easily accessible on your phone). This is one of my favorite exercises to start the day in a positive light, and it comes from Pam Grout's book, *E*[3] (E cube). It is a straightforward and quick exercise that only takes a few minutes.

  - "Happy" by Pharrell Williams.
  - "What a Wonderful World" by Louis Armstrong
  - "Best Day of My Life" by American Authors
  - "I Believe I Can Fly" by R. Kelly
  - "Three Little Birds" by Bob Marley
  - "Celebration" by Kool and the Gang
  - "I Feel Good" by James Brown
  - "I Gotta a Feeling" by Black-eyed Peas
  - "Seasons of Love" from the *Rent* soundtrack

  Pump your fist in the air with complete glee (five times). Do the Harlem Shuffle on the way to the bathroom before you brush your teeth. Notice all these songs have positive lyrics about the world and encourage good feelings. What an excellent way to start the day! Hey, why not challenge yourself and, instead of listening to one of these songs, listen to all of them first thing in the morning?

Remember, true happiness and inner peace are not automatic. Authentic lasting happiness and inner peace come from making a conscious choice to be happy on a consistent basis, regardless of the circumstances that surround us. Therefore, by performing one or two intentional activities daily, such as the ones mentioned above, you can make improvements in your enduring levels of happiness and overcome hedonic adaptation.

You can't wait for external conditions to change before you allow yourself to feel happy. You must proactively move toward the vision of the person you want to be and the feelings you want to experience. Therefore, it is not enough to do these activities on days that things are not going your way or you are upset. Instead create a daily practice that generates these positive thoughts, feelings, and high vibrations, and with time, these will become your new habits.

This is important because your habits are what create your character, and your character is what determines your destiny. More importantly, consciously choosing to be happy will empower you to take control over your life because you will stop relying on external circumstances, material things, food, and other people to be happy.

These activities do not have to take too much time out of your day. I follow a very simple practice that I have found effective:

- First thing in the morning when I wake up, I take ten to fifteen minutes to go over my goals, affirmations, and visualizations. I do this regardless of what is going on in my life. For example, on some days, I must get my kid ready for school. Or I have special meetings, make breakfast, go to work, prepare lunches, and so on. How I make this work is by simply planning to wake up fifteen minutes before the activities of that specific day are scheduled to start. I may also read a book in the morning. It will depend on how busy the day is going to be.

- While I shower and get dressed, I listen to songs with positive lyrics (listed above).

- I listen to a lecture or a positive book on my drive to and from work.

- When I arrive into the office, I make tea and take time to write three things that I am grateful for and three things that I am looking forward to. I also plan my day. (Panda Planner is a great resource for this activity.)

- At lunchtime, I take a thirty-minute walk. During this walk, I listen to positive affirmations on my phone. Not only does this activity break up my day and help me be more productive, it also promotes emotional and physical health.

- After dinner, if I did not have an opportunity to read in the morning, I read a positive or inspiring book for at least twenty minutes.
- At the end of the day (ten to fifteen minutes before I go to bed), I review my day, list what went well and what can I do to improve, and meditate.

It sounds like there is a lot of time involved, but if you look carefully, the actual extra time that I am taking out of my day for these activities adds up to only about an hour. The rest of the activities are integrated into my regular daily tasks, for example, listening to a book while I drive to work. Depending on your lifestyle your daily practice may look very different. What is important is to be specific and clear of what tasks you are going to incorporate into your life and schedule them into your day. If they are not planned, they most likely won't get done. Because you will get distracted by the many competing tasks, demands, issues, and other priorities in your life.

Additionally, do not wait for inspiration to hit you before you do these activities. Otherwise, you will hear yourself making excuses such as, "I deserve a break", "I had a long day", "I'm too busy", "I'm tired", "The house is too messy". Instead, act like these activities are part of your daily responsibilities, for example your job or kids and get them done.

In order to successfully implement these changes, when getting started don't overdo it. I did not build this schedule all at once. Instead, I added tasks over time. This is about building wellness habits. Therefore, start by introducing one item into your life, once you are comfortable add another one, even if you feel you are going too slow, it is ok. What we are looking for is progress.

Remember, no matter how busy you are you can choose to spare an hour a day for personal development. It is your life, and your daily choices create it.

NATURAL SUPPLEMENTS TO SUPPORT EMOTIONAL HEALTH

We all have times in our lives when we need a little support from external sources such as herbs to help us cope with a stressful or difficult event(s) in our lives. In such times, you can use herbs and flower essences to help you manage stress, anxiety, and other emotions while you work on correcting the physical and emotional imbalance in your body and mind. Such was the case with my son. He took herbs and flower essence in a time in his life when he was suffering from severe depression:

> At age fourteen, my son was diagnosed with severe depression and was suicidal. He felt hopeless and angry. And since he was not improving much with counseling alone, his psychiatrist felt the only solution was to medicate him with psychotropics, which I was willing to try if and only if we were unable to correct the issue with diet, exercise, counseling, and an herbal supplement. Therefore, I spoke with his psychologist, and we came up with a plan. I created an herbal formula based on his apparent symptoms and a tongue assessment (Chinese medicine diagnosis technique). This herbal formula included antidepressant herbs such as St. John's wort and rhodiola as well as hawthorn, an herb known to calm the heart and the spirit. It also included cleansing and hormone-balancing herbs. (Since he was a teen, hormones could be a part of the issue.) Lastly, I added herbs to clear heat (fire element) because his tongue showed a lot of heat in the body, and we also know that ups and downs in emotions are usually related to fire element.
>
> The second formula created for him was a flower essence to help restore hope and self-love and increase motivation. He went on a diet as described in chapter 9, took an omega-3, -6, and -9 supplement. Within a week of starting this protocol, we began to see a difference in his mood and behavior. By the four-week mark, he was acting like his old self again. This change in behavior allowed him to be more open and receptive during his counseling sessions, which in turn helped him recover faster. His counseling was well rounded. He went three times per week and included group and individual therapy (DBT), art, music, and meditation therapy as well. He also worked with affirmations and visualization.

Now my son is healthy and without any issues, and we did it all with traditional medicine therapies that supported the mind, body, and his spirit. Please note that my son was in an outpatient treatment center and was under constant supervision to make sure he did not hurt himself while we tried this approach. Therefore, make sure you have the appropriate support before you try this on a suicidal person.

Nervine and adaptogen herbs are nutritive and directly benefit the nervous system. Moreover, herbal nervine therapy increases our ability to cope with the stress of daily life. You may take nervines and adaptogen herbs as you need them. However, if you are under chronic stress, you may benefit from taking nerve tonic herbs on a regular basis such as:

HERB	HEALTH BENEFITS
California poppy	This herb has been used as an anti-anxiety and sedative. It helps with insomnia, nerve pain, aches, ADHD, and improved cognitive function.
Catnip	This diaphoretic herb relieves anxiety and stress, helps with restless sleep, soothes menstrual pain, and eases stomach discomfort such as gas. It reduces pain and is a sedative.
Chamomile	It is anti-anxiety and works for depression. It is fights allergy fighter or treats hay fever. It is an anti-inflammatory and treats muscle spasms, PMS and other menstrual disorders, insomnia, skin disorders, ulcers, wounds, and gastrointestinal disorders. It is an arthritis and rheumatic cure. It is a pain reliever and treats hemorrhoids, amongst many others
Hops	Hops promotes sleep and reduces menopausal symptoms. It is antiviral, anti-clotting, anti-inflammatory, and antitumor. It may protect against cell damage that causes Alzheimer's and Parkinson's.
Lavender	One of the most common herbs used, it's a powerful antioxidant. It is antimicrobial, sedative, calming, and antidepressant. Additionally it is used to relieve anxiety and stress, protect against diabetes, improve cognitive function, heal burns and wounds, improve sleep, improve skin complexion and reduce acne, relieve pain, and alleviate headaches.

Lemon Balm	Lemon balm is antibacterial. It improves sleep reduces anxiety, heals wounds, protects the liver against cancer cells, lowers triglycerides, reduces blood sugar, helps treat the herpes virus, and improves cognitive function, mood, concentration, and sleep.
Oat Straw	Oat straw is high in calcium and other minerals, protein, and the spectrum of B vitamins, except vitamin B-12. Oat straw is also high in silica, a mineral that is mainly responsible for healthy skin, hair, nails, and bones. It has also been used for broken bones and sexual dysfunction. It soothes and nourishes the central nervous system. Therefore, it treats anxiety, insomnia, and nervousness.
Passion Flower	It has been used to reduce and eliminate insomnia, anxiety, inflammation from skin irritations and burns, menopause symptoms, ADHD, seizures, high blood pressure, and asthma.
Skullcap	This herb has been used for anxiety, insomnia, and inflammation. It provides relief from spasms, stimulates blood flow in the pelvic region, encourages menstruation, helps eliminate headaches, reduces fever, treats gout, and works as a sedative.
St. John's wort	Most famous for its antidepressant and anti-inflammatory properties, this herb can also be used for nerve pain, anxiety, tiredness, loss of appetite and trouble sleeping, ADHD, OCD, seasonal affective disorder (SAD), and symptoms of menopause.
Valerian	It eases insomnia, anxiety, and nervous restlessness. It is also antispasmodic, relieves nerve pain, lowers blood pressure, and relieves menstrual cramps.
Wood Betony	This herb helps with headaches, muscle aches, and nerve pain. It opens the lungs and releases tension, stress, and anxiety. Wood betony has a slow and mild effect that accumulates over time.

You can also manage stress and other negative emotions with flower essences. Flower essences are not to be confused with aromatherapy (essential oils) they are infusions made from the flowering part of a plant. Every flower has a different healing quality, and because each flower acts as an agent of change at a deep emotional level, they offer an excellent way to heal and grow. Some of the positive changes that flower essences can help you include feeling more positive, confident, and creative, experiencing more joy, love, and peace, being more forgiving and accepting, forming better relationships, and having more clarity, focus, and concentration, amongst many others.

Flower essences will begin working in a matter of seconds, minutes, or days. It will depend on the situation, person, and depth of the issue. Also the change may be very noticeable or subtle, with changes occurring over time. Nevertheless, because they trigger the body to rebalance an emotional state that is out of balance, they will have a long-term effect. In times where the imbalance remains, there is usually something external that needs to change such as a job or a relationship, and sometimes flower essence serve as a catalyst or inspiration to make this change but is up to you to act.

There are literally hundreds of flower essences. You can start with experimenting with the Bach flower essences or the California flower essences. Both can be found online with a description of how each flower can assist you. You can also use the flower essences that I designed specifically for this program. You can find it on my website at https://www.moongazingapothecary.com/autoimmune-herbal-supplements.htm

Essential oils are also an excellent alternative to manage negative emotions, such as stress, anxiety, sadness, and depression. Some of my favorite essential oils for promoting positive feelings are:

EMOTION	ESSENTIAL OIL
Sadness/uplifting	Clary sage, lemon, tangerine, lime, bergamot, peppermint
Unfocused	Basil, peppermint, rosemary
Tiredness	Orange, peppermint, frankincense
Forgetfulness	Rosemary, peppermint
Anger, frustration, and tension	Lavender, ylang, ylang, petitgrain, Roman chamomile, bergamot
Worry and anxiousness	Chamomile, bergamot, lavender, jasmine, neroli, helichrysum, rose, nutmeg

Depression	Neroli, Roman and German chamomiles, helichrysum, spikenard, lavender, rose
Promote positive mood	Jasmine, ylang ylang, rosemary, patchouli, melissa, coriander, marjoram, frankincense, myrrh, vetiver, clary sage, cypress, gucalyptus globulus, hyssop, pine needle, tea tree, ginger, geranium, juniper berry
Insomnia	Lavender, nutmeg, vetiver, chamomile, ylang ylang, bergamot, sandalwood, marjoram, cerdarwood, frankincense

There are many ways to enjoy the benefits from essential oils, including but not limited to:

- Diffuse essential oils with a room diffuser or a car diffuser while you are on the road.
- Use scent balls in smaller rooms.
- Use a personal inhaler and inhale a few whiffs every now and again.
- Add them to massage oils.
- Add a few drops to bath water.
- Create oil-based perfumes with a carrier oil
- Create an essential oil spray by adding witch hazel or water to a glass spray bottle and a few drops of the essential oil(s) of your choice.
- Apply one or two drops to jewelry.

Select the appropriate oils for your current condition and make your own essential oil blend, or you can also use the essential oil blends that I designed specifically for this program. You can find it on my website at https://www.moongazingapothecary.com/autoimmune-herbal-supplements.html.

Also this is a basic anti-anxiety and sleep aid essential oil formula that you can create at home. Not only does this spice blend have a fresh-baked pumpkin pie scent, it will also help you relax and disinfect the air. It is also a great substitute to those synthetically perfumed candles.

PUMPKIN SPICE AROMA ESSENTIAL OIL BLEND

- Twenty drops cinnamon EO
- Twenty drops ginger EO
- Twenty drops nutmeg EO
- Fifteen drops clove bud EO
- Five drops cardamom EO

Add all essential oils to a glass bottle. One one-quarter ounce bottle will hold this blend perfectly. Screw cap on tightly, and invert the bottle to blend the oils.

Diffusing: Fill your essential oil diffuser reservoir with water. Add five to six drops of the Pumpkin Spice Essential Oil Blend. Light a tea candle in the base of your diffuser and enjoy as your space fills with this spicy aroma!

Another essential nutrient that has a positive effect on our mental health is omega-3 oil and other omega oils. Omega oil has an incredible impact on our brain, especially when it comes to mild memory loss and depression. Additionally, omega oils are a potent anti-inflammatory, and they support heart health. Moreover, clinical studies concluded that taking omega oils such as the ones found in fish oil supplements improved depression symptoms, with effects comparable to those of antidepressant medications. There are vegan options for this supplement, one being UDOs oil.

As you can see, there are many options (methods) that can help you stay positive and focused as you go about your day. Use one or as many as you need throughout your day.

ADRENAL GLAND SUPPORT

In addition to managing your stress, if you suffer from an autoimmune disorder, a chronic illness, or chronic stress, it will be essential for you to support your nervous system and adrenal glands with adaptogen herbs such as the ones described in chapter 10. Reason being constant exposure to emotional stress and trauma, chronic illness and pain, inefficient sleep, toxins, and a poor diet may cause adrenal fatigue or in general affect your central nervous system. Overactive adrenals produce too much cortisol, epinephrine (adrenaline) and aldosterone, which can lead to insulin resistance and metabolic syndrome.

Simply stated, adrenal fatigue is the inability of your adrenal glands to cope with stress. More importantly, when you have adrenal fatigue, every organ and system in your body is significantly affected, and changes occur in your carbohydrate, protein, and fat metabolism, fluid and electrolyte balance, and reproductive and cardiovascular system. Moreover, adrenal fatigue and every occurrence of significant stress, anger, grief, sadness, lifestyle change, or another high stimulus can also severly burden the thyroid. Therefore, the adrenal function must be corrected before they thyroid gland can function adequetly. Note that weak adrenals can cause hypothyroid symptoms, even when the thyroid itself does not show any deficiencies in lab tests.

The symptoms of adrenal fatigue include but are not limited to[91] chronic fatigue, trouble getting to sleep and waking up, salt and sugar cravings, food sensitivities, unexplained weight gain or loss, reliance on stimulants such as caffeine, light-headedness, loss of body hair and skin discoloration, autoimmune conditions, brain fog, hormone imbalance, weakened anxiety and stress response, insulin resistance, decreased libido, moodiness, anger and irritability, depression, muscle or bone loss, chronic infections, hair loss, water retention, weakness in the legs and skin conditions.

The topic or diagnosis of adrenal fatigue or any other disorder is beyond the scope of this book. If you need more information on adrenal fatigue, I recommend James Wilson's book, *Adrenal Fatigue—The 21st Century Stress Syndrome.* Even if you are not suffering from adrenal fatigue or if you have an autoimmune disorder, a chronic illness, or chronic stress, as part of this program, it will be essential for you to support your nervous system and adrenal glands with adaptogen herbs such as the ones described in chapter 10.

NUTRITIONAL RECOMMENDATIONS FOR THE ADRENALS

Adequate nutrition through diet is critical for good functioning of the adrenals. Foods and supplements that are beneficial for the adrenal glands include those rich in fatty acids (see chapter nine for more information), antioxidants, vitamin C, E, and all B vitamins, magnesium, zinc, L-thyroisne, phosphytidylserine, and adaptogen herbs.

Adaptogens are substances that help the body better cope with mental, environmental, and physical stress, support metabolic functions, and help restore balance. According to David Winston and Steven Maimes, adaptogens are unique from other herbs in their ability to restore the balance of endocrine hormones, modulate the immune system, and allow the body to maintain optimal homeostasis.[92]

To qualify as an adaptogen, an herb must be safe and nontoxic; must have broad uses for health and specifically reduce mental, physical, and environmental stress; and has a normalizing effect on physiology, irrespective of the direction of change caused by physiological norms created by the stressor.[92]

You can create your own using the herbs mentioned in chapter 8. Or you can use the herbal adaptogen formula that I designed specifically for this program. You can find it on my website at https://www.moongazingapothecary.com/autoimmune-herbal-supplements.htm. Or drink the chai maca tea daily mentioned in chapter 9. (You may substitute maca with a different adaptogen like reishi.)

Additionally people who are under chronic stress are often deficient in vitamins B and C. This deficiency can impact your health. There is a strong correlation between low levels of vitamin B-12 to muscle weakness, lack of coordination, and even loss of muscle mass. Moreover, when you are a B-12 deficient, your body can't accurately convert carbohydrates into glucose that is useable throughout the body. Since your body uses glucose for energy, without it, you will feel tired. Consuming the right food like the diet in chapter 9 should be enough for you to get sufficient vitamin B. However if you are not getting enough nutrients from your diet and if you are under chronic stress, it is recommended that you take vitamin B and C supplements.

MINDFULNESS IMPROVES HEALTH AND MINIMIZES STRESS AND OTHER NEGATIVE EMOTIONS

"The present moment is filled with joy and happiness. If you are attentive, you will see it," said Thich Nhat Hanh.

Another technique to improve mental health is mindfulness. Studies have shown that mindfulness has many health benefits, including reducing stress and enhancing your ability to deal with everyday struggles. Additionally, when you reach a state of relaxation like the one achieved with mindfulness, you can reap the following benefits: higher brain and cognitive function such as increased clarity in thinking and perception as well as increased focus and attention, increased immune function, lowered blood pressure and heart rate, increased awareness, lowered anxiety levels, feeling calm and internally still, feeling connected, and decreased depression symptoms.

Mindfulness has been shown to increase coping mechanisms in cancer and other terminal illness patients as well as reduce symptoms. A study on mindfulness in college students found that medical and psychology students who practiced mindfulness reported improvements in many areas, such as decreased reactivity, increased curiosity and affected tolerance, improved patience and self-acceptance, and enhanced relational qualities.[93]

Mindfulness in children found that mindfulness improved emotion regulation, mood, empathy, confidence, and self-esteem as well as coping and social skills and their ability to pay attention and focus.[94] Mindfulness was shown to boost resilience in children and help them understand and regulate their own emotions.[93] Mindfulness-based cognitive therapy for children reduces behavioral and attention problems and anxiety.[95]

Furthermore, there are a broad number of studies on the effectiveness of mindfulness and meditation in the areas of stress reduction, increased productivity at work, enhanced brain function, improved academic success, reduced alcohol consumption, and improved general health, amongst many others. Therefore, everyone has something to gain from practicing mindfulness.

However, to reap maximum benefits, it must occur regularly and often. To start seeing results, you need to practice daily for ten minutes at least for five to eight weeks. The good news is there are many ways to apply mindfulness in your everyday life. Include something as simple of just closing your eyes and being silent for a few minutes a day.

Moreover, there are hundreds of mindfulness practices available to you. One of the most common is practicing mindful, focused breathing. Slow, deep, rhythmic breathing causes stimulation of the parasympathetic nervous system, which results in a reduction in the heart rate and relaxation of muscles. (See appendix B for an example.)

As you can see, the benefits of mindfulness are vast, and whether or not you suffer from chronic stress, anxiety, or any other negative emotions, you will benefit greatly from taking on a mindfulness practice. For more exercises on mindfulness, see part one of appendix E

COGNITIVE RESTRUCTURING: CHANGE YOUR THOUGHTS; CHANGE YOUR LIFE

"You mainly feel the way you think," said Albert Ellis.

Another highly effective strategy to manage your emotions is cognitive restructuring. As with mindfulness, the basis for this technique is the concept that all pain is caused by our thoughts and our interpretation of the events that are happening in our lives, rather than the inherent situation. As Dr. Wayne Dyer used to point out, "There is no such thing as stress, there are only people thinking stressful thoughts."

I believe that this concept can apply to any other emotion. After all, our lives are just an endless sequence of events and thoughts about those events.

Therefore, happiness and all other positive emotions are already in your consciousness, but your limiting beliefs and negative emotional patterns are just concealing them.

Needless thoughts in the form of dysfunctional beliefs are like any other bad habit. They automatically occur. We don't even notice them, and they are often the root cause of all negative emotions and experiences. It is true that we often can't change the situation or event that is causing us stress or distress, but we can change our response to it. Our responses come from our thoughts, and our thoughts come from a belief. However, "It is only a thought, and a thought can be changed," as Louise Hay used to say.

So how do we change our thoughts and beliefs? The answer is with mindfulness and cognitive restructuring. Psychotherapists commonly use this technique to teach people how to react to events differently. This technique involves learning to recognize negative thoughts as they come up and change them so we can become more realistic in our thinking regarding the event that is causing us stress; see the event more clearly; reduce tunnel vision that often comes while you are under stress; and minimize false alarms that sometimes show up when we are under stress.

Cognitive restructuring is a potent therapy technique. However, one disadvantage of this technique is that it is sometimes difficult for people to learn without the assistance of a therapist. This is because sometimes the stories we tell ourselves are like autosuggestions that hypnotize us and make it hard for us to see that other possibilities exists. Therefore, we often aren't able to identify the cognitive distortion that is causing distress, or we are focused on justifying (reasoning) the way we think. It is also very common for people to believe they are doing the technique right when they are not and incorrectly conclude that the method does not work. Nevertheless, here is one exercise that you can try on your own:

1. The first step is to become aware of negative thoughts. This is one of the most challenging parts of the exercise because negative thoughts tend to be automatic. You can do this by monitoring and recording events during the day that caused you to stress. Write them down.

2. Once you have time to do this exercise (maybe at the end of the day), review the situation and think about what thoughts when through your mind during this event. Write them down. Look for distortions or dysfunctional beliefs. Do certain conditions trigger negative thought patterns? Are you a black-and-white thinker in specific topics? Do you typically experience anger or sadness in response to stress?

3. The next step is to reframe the negative thoughts by writing down more accurate, adaptive thoughts about the event. This is not always easy, but these questions can help you:

    a. Are my thoughts on the event correct?

    b. Am I using words such as *never, always, worst, terrible,* or *horrible* to describe the event?

    c. What objective evidence or facts exist to support my view? In other words, what evidence do I have that this situation will turn out this way?

    d. Am I overemphasizing a negative aspect of this event or person?

    e. What positive alternative views are there for the event?

    f. Am I catastrophizing, awfulizing, jumping to conclusions, and assuming an adverse outcome?

    g. Is there anything positive about this situation?

    h. Am I undervaluing my ability to cope with the event?

    i. How much will this matter next week, in a month, or year?

    j. If I had one month to live, how important will this be?

    k. What is the worst that can happen if my view of the event is correct?

    l. What actions can I take to influence the event?

    m. What is the worst thing that could happen to my family or me, and how does this event compare to that?

4. After thinking things through, restate your original beliefs regarding the event so they are more realistic and less distorted. You can do this by rewriting your original thought. Write down new positive ways of thinking or more helpful beliefs that direct to a new approach to deal with the event. It will take time and practice, but in time, you will be able to start changing the nonhelpful stress-inducing thoughts as they come, and you will find yourself feeling less stress and therefore happier.

If you are interested in learning cognitive restructuring, I recommend that, in the beginning, you work with an experienced cognitive behavioral or compassion focus therapist that can assist and teach you how to recognize negative thoughts and reframe them. You can do this over the course of six to ten weekly sessions. Once you get the hang of the method, you can work on it on your own. If you want to try it on your own, I have found Byron Katie's books extremely helpful and easy for learning cognitive restructuring, in particular, the book *Loving What Is*. You can also practice on your own the "feeling exercise" from Arnold Patent (appendix E).

Finally, it is essential to be patient and kind to yourself while you are implementing changes related to the way your brain has been trained to process the world. Understand that your old habits will keep persistently reasserting themselves. There is a neurological reason for this, your habits have created well-established neuropathways conditioned to fire off in certain situations. Additionally, pain and negative emotions activate the reward centers of the brain, such as the beta-endorphin and dopamine pathways, causing unconscious addiction to pain and negative emotions like self-pity, anger, stress, and guilt.

Yes! You read correctly! We can be addicted to our negative emotions. Therefore, unless you are putting effort and intention to change on a consistent basis, those neuropathways will pull you back to your old ways of thinking and behaving. This is why it is common to regress or have setbacks while you are in the process of making changes. However, don't get discouraged and try and try again. Change does not happen overnight. This means you can't just do an exercise here and there. If you want lasting results, you must be consistent, create new habits, and redesign the nine environments covered in chapter 5 to support these changes.

Even though change takes time, it is not impossible. Research has shown that it takes between twenty-six and thirty days to build new neuropathways, in other words, "rewire" the brain. And a study by Phillipa Lally demonstrated that, on average, it takes two months before a new behavior becomes automatic, sixty-six days to be exact.[96] And this can vary widely depending on the action, the person, and the circumstances. Habits are important because you become your habits. Therefore, the habits you choose to create will set the tone for your entire life. Choose wisely.

Moreover, it is important to note that it is not just our thoughts and beliefs that shape our reality. It is also our actions. When we take steps to change, we stimulate our consciousness and help accelerate the creation of new beliefs and habits, so regardless of setbacks, don't give up. It is ok to get help. You do not have to do this alone. You can do this work in groups or with a coach or a mentor, an accountability partner, or a friend.

Remember, pain is a choice; an expression of your free will. So the question is: Do you love yourself enough to give yourself the gift of joy?

CHAPTER THIRTEEN

Self-Love – The Heart of Healing

You yourself, as much as anybody in the entire universe, deserve your love and affection.

—BUDDHA

Self-love is a necessary part of health and well-being, and it encompasses self-compassion, self-care, and self-forgiveness. Love is a positive energy that is necessary for a healthy balance among mind, body, and spirit. In fact, to be healthy, it is essential to have a healthy sense of self-esteem and self-love. People who genuinely love themselves care about what they are eating, create healthy boundaries in their relationships, have great self-control, and make choices with intention. In other words, they ask themselves, "Is this good for me?" before making any decisions on what they eat, whom they spend time with, and what is in the environments that surround them.

For this reason, self-love means you wholeheartedly love and accept yourself, regardless of how you look, feel, or act, and you make yourself and your needs a priority. It does not include pushing yourself to the limits, putting someone's needs above your own, and wishing that "someday" you will have time to take care of yourself and do what you love. It is important to note that self-love is not at all about being self-centered in a selfish, "all about me" way.

Instead it's about honoring our feelings, taking time for ourselves, and caring for ourselves in the same way we care for others. Unfortunately, for the most part, most people are unaware that they lack self-love and that their lives are controlled and regulated by negative images and attitudes toward themselves.[97] Let's look at some of the indications that a person lacks self-love. (You may experience one or many of this signs.)

- You are quick to criticize yourself.
- You choose to believe you are unlovable.
- You are continually justifying why you do love yourself.
- You are afraid to charge an appropriate amount for your services.
- You are sensitive to criticism.
- You are indecisive in a way that keeps people reacting to your new choices and therefore receiving their attention and energy.
- You exhibit social withdrawal.
- You convince yourself and maybe others that your irrational anxiety is just part of your personality or is about what is going on in your life instead of taking responsibility for creating the life you are living.
- You express hostility.
- You judge other people for small, subjective, arbitrary things.
- You have an excessive preoccupation with personal problems and are overwhelmed with crises in your life.
- You have a compulsive need to micromanage your home and bodies. You blame it on OCD and so on.

- You continuously experience physical symptoms such as fatigue, insomnia, pain, and headaches.
- You don't take care of your body because "other things are more important."
- You live in chaos or disorder.
- You settle for something you don't want, but you justify the reason and don't call it "settling."
- You place other people's needs above your own so often that you are worn out.
- You keep going back to the things that hurt you and the people who don't want you.
- You spend sleepless nights replaying dramas that you wish you'd handled differently and inwardly berate yourself for being so "stupid" and "thoughtless."
- You have an unhealthy compulsion to repeatedly think about past events and mull them over (rumination).
- You tend to make your emotional pain worse by turning to addictions like alcohol, sugar, drugs, and so on.
- You consistently spend money or create debt.[98, 99]
- You are continually comparing yourself to others.
- You are not honest with your emotions or blame others. (You play the victim.)
- You do not follow your heart or follow your true path in life.
- You keep people who you don't like in your life.
- You feel as if bad things always happen to you, and you can never figure out why you have seemingly unfair misfortune.

In any situation, you can always measure of how much love you are feeling or withholding from yourself by the degree of comfort or discomfort you are currently feeling. Discomfort is a signal that you are withholding love. Therefore, underneath almost all our suffering and illness lies a lack of self-compassion and self-care. For instance, poor lifestyle choices, such as smoking, overuse of alcohol, poor diet, lack of physical activity, and inadequate relief of chronic stress have been linked to be key contributors in the development and progression of preventable chronic diseases, including obesity, type 2 diabetes mellitus, hypertension, cardiovascular disease, autoimmune diseases, and several types of cancer. It is important to note that the withholding of love in many occasions started years earlier, and it often begins in childhood when you interpreted the actions of a particular individual towards you as unloving or unsupportive. This interpretation or judgment results in a constraint of energy in your body, which is experienced as discomfort. Forgiveness is the key to releasing the energy that has been locked up by our perceptions and judgments.

We are also, on an unconscious level, continually attracting to us people and relationships that reflect a part of ourselves that we do not entirely love and accept. Therefore, every single relationship in our lives reflects an aspect of our ourselves. When we truly love ourselves, we attract loving, peaceful relationships. On the other hand, a person in our lives who brings up unpleasant feelings in us, you can be sure is someone, or represents someone from our past, that we have not forgiven and are ready to forgive.

Consequently, everyone that we attract into our lives is there to help us learn to love ourselves and come to peace with our past by taking on the roles of family members and other authority figures from our childhood whom we are ready to forgive. As you come to genuinely to love and accept these people as they are and for the role they are playing in your life, you will make peace with the part of yourself that the individual is reflecting.

In the end, the person you are really forgiving is yourself. That is because when you release your interpretations or judgments towards another, you are really freeing yourself from the perceptions of yourself, and it is in actuality a gift of self-love.

In addition to forgiving, having compassion for yourself is as important as having compassion for others. There is evidence that harsh self-criticism and lack of self-esteem activates the sympathetic nervous system, in other words, fight-or-flight response. Therefore, they elevate stress hormones such as cortisol in our bloodstream. Furthermore, if you are constantly judging, criticizing yourself, or comparing yourself to others, you are creating artificial boundaries that will lead to feelings of separation and isolation.

On the other hand, having high self-esteem doesn't just feel good, it has physical benefits too. It seems that self-esteem protects the heart and immune system.[98] Moreover, aside from keeping you healthy, self-love can also make you feel good and can benefit your life in other ways too, for example:

- Higher life satisfaction is often correlated with people who practice self-love. Appreciating yourself helps you appreciate your life and motivates you to work toward fulfilling your purpose in life. You also tend to have more enjoyment and a more positive attitude toward the future.
- Self-love decreases stress, lessens procrastination, and reduces performance anxiety around deadlines, consequently increasing performance.
- Self-love can drive you to adopt healthy habits and take care of your physical self.
- People who practice self-love rebound from adversity faster than those who wallow in self-loathing. It is a fact that we can't control what life throws at us, but we can manage our response to each of the events in our lives. People who feel good about themselves handle life crises better and move on to the good times faster.
- Self-love promotes better mental health because it can keep you from getting lost in your head and going down a path toward ruminating on negative thoughts and feelings.
- Those who have confidence and self-love tend to behave in ways that allow them to be more successful and happy. They also are more likely to take advantage of opportunities that will make them more money. Additionally they will look toward their past achievements to know that they can succeed in new

> financial efforts. On the other hand, people with low self-esteem and negative thinking patterns tend to sabotage their chances of financial success by looking at past failures to justify their negative self-image, thereby hindering their economic growth.

Research from Dr. Paul Gilbert and others have demonstrated that self-compassion is a powerful way to achieve self-love, emotional well-being, and contentment in our lives. According to Kristen Neff, PhD, the definition of self-compassion is very similar to that of compassion for others.

> Self-compassion involves wanting health and wellbeing for oneself and *leads to proactive behavior* to better one's situation rather than passivity. And self-compassion does not mean that I think my problems are more important than yours, it just means that I think my problems are *also* important and worthy of being attended to … Love, connection, and acceptance are your birth right. To claim them need only look within yourself.[99]

Because self-love is a loving attitude from which positive actions arise that benefit you and others, many experts believe that learning to be kind to yourself is the foundation of kindness to others. However, they state that true benevolence is felt directly by the heart, and it transcends any egoistic accounting of an individual's apparent good actions. Also because compassion is a state of mind or the heart, it cannot be measured by a person's outward behaviors. And people who exhaust themselves doing things for others out of a desire to be liked or out of fear that others will get angry at them are not experiencing healthy compassion.[43] Therefore, an individual will not benefit from this type of experience. This has been observed clearly in studies examining changes in volunteers over time. These studies have demonstrated that it is only when it is not too burdensome that helping others has benefits for the helper.[13]

Moreover, according to Ladner, if an individual is feeling stressed out, overwhelmed, or unhappy while helping others, he or she has not been experiencing genuine compassion because the unconscious essence of stress is a heart that is closed off from others in an inner world of agitated, fearful thoughts and feelings. Consequently these feelings block a person from developing genuine compassion. It is critical that people approach compassion practically, beginning by assessing how much they can do for others without feeling stressed out, overwhelmed, or depleted.[43]

Likewise, healthy boundaries are vital for maintaining a sense of self-respect. Setting healthy limits includes saying no or refusing to do something or interact in a certain way when not refusing likely would lead people to feel stressed out, hurt, disrespected, resentful, and/or angry. Setting healthy boundaries works directly against negative patterns, like the compulsive desire to be liked or tendency not to take care of ourselves or to be cruel to ourselves. As a result, setting boundaries involves being honest and direct with others, even if they don't want to hear what needs to be said.

In conclusion, not only is loving yourself good for your overall health and happiness, it is also good for everyone around you. It creates the kind of joy you bring with you wherever you go, and by radiating this happy, joyful energy toward the planet, you will contribute to the shift of the earth from instability and discord to one of balance, cooperation, and peace. Michio Kushi relates,

We all come from infinity,
We all live within infinity,
We all shall return to infinity,
We are all manifestation of one infinity,
We are all brothers and sisters of one infinite universe,
Let us love each other,
Let us help each other,
Let us encourage each other,
Let us all continue to realize the endless dream of one peaceful world,
We are always one forever.

RESOURCES TO LEARN HOW TO LOVE YOURSELF

There are many books, therapists, and teachers that can help you take steps to learn to love yourself, and I will cover a couple of techniques in part four of this book, However, this is a list of resources and actions that can serve you as a guide:

- Be kind to yourself. Quiet the inner critic that judges your actions and feelings.
- Make decisions from a place of love instead of fear.
- Express gratitude for what you have each day.
- Don't compare yourself to others.
- Grape flower essence works great to help increase qualities of love and devotion such as realization of the inner source of love (self-love); loving without condition, demand, or expectation; patience with others' shortcomings; and healthy sexuality.
- Practice writing self-love affirmations twenty-nine times every day.
- Become mindful of your thoughts, feelings, and wants.
- Practice emotional freedom technique (EFT). You can search on the internet for videos that can teach you how to do EFT or read the book, *The Tapping Solution*, from Nick Orton.
- Practice compassion focus therapy.
- Practice forgiveness of the self and others. (For exercises to help you forgive, see appendix D and E).
- Read books on self-love:
    - Any book from Louise Hay, in particular, *You Can Heal Your Life*
    - *Loveability* and *Shift Happens* from Robert Holden
    - *May Cause Miracles* by Gabrielle Bernstein
    - *Life Loves You* from Robert Holden and Louise Hay
    - *Loving What Is* by Byron Katie

It has been said by many masters and it has also been my experience that, when you believe you are worthy, your life will reflect it. This is because the way we see ourselves and, more importantly, the way we feel about ourselves determines how we experience life. When people start to love themselves, their lives begin to change for the better, and they begin to create positive circumstances that reflect their self-love. Their mood improves. Consequently, they start attracting good things into their lives. For example, they get the job they were asking for, they find the home of their dreams, the money they need shows up, relationships improve, and new ones form. However, it is important to note that when people make a positive change in their self-image, they also tend to become anxious because the shift marks a separation from the identity they formed in childhood.[97] According to Robert W. Firestone, Ph.D., "This separation appears to be related symbolically to breaking the fantasy bond, an imagined connection with their parent or primary caregiver, which arouses feelings of sadness, guilt, and anxiety."

Therefore, it is imperative that you are kind and patient with yourself when making these changes. Take it a day at a time, and do not judge or criticize yourself if you take a step back during this process. In other words, love yourself through the process.

PART FOUR

Putting All Together – 12 Week Protocol To Health

Being healthy and fit is not a fad or a trend. Instead, it is a lifestyle

---

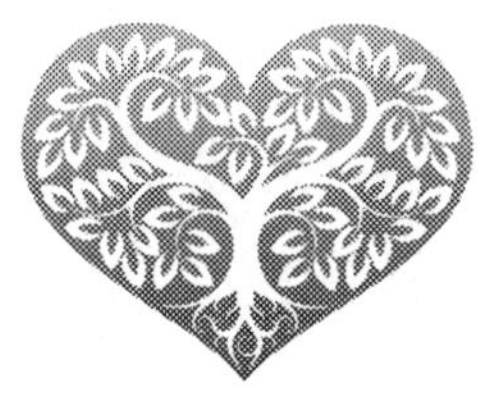

CHAPTER FOURTEEN

12-Week Step by Step Program to Health

You are not your illness. You have an individual story to tell. You have a name, a history, a personality. Staying yourself is part of the battle.

—JULIAN SEIFTER

This section of the book is where you will be applying all the concepts you have learned throughout this book. I will lead you through this program step-by-step, explaining the changes you will need to implement each week. During this program, I will be asking you to introduce into your life the diet, breathing exercises, and changes to your environment discussed earlier in this book. I will also present at the appropriate time frame the herbal supplements that you can use to help you restore your body. Throughout this program, you will also learn how you can change long-standing patterns of behavior that may be causing your health problems.

The twelve-week program consists of small changes that build upon each other, and by the end of this program, you will have laid the foundation for well-being. Then you can then decide what works for you and how much of the program you want to keep on a permanent basis. So let's get started!

Note that this program is not intended to be a substitute for the care of a licensed medical doctor. I strongly advise you to seek the advice of your physician or qualified health care practitioner before starting this program or changing current medical treatment. Any information or herbal supplement mentioned in this book is not intended to be a substitute for professional medical advice.

WEEK 1

It is essential to make a priority to strengthen and rebuild your body. Therefore, the focus of week one is to start cleansing and nourishing your body.

1. If you have any symptoms that are currently bothering you, such as stress, headaches, pain, or high blood pressure, it is vital that you continue managing those symptoms as you are now doing. However, whenever possible, substitute any toxic medications with herbs and supplements. For example, if you suffer from headaches, instead of Tylenol, try an herbal supplement designed for those symptoms like meadowsweet or willow bark.

2. Start an herbal detox supplement. You can use the herbal cleansing formula that I designed specifically for this program. You can find it on my website at https://www.moongazingapothecary.com/autoimmune-herbal-supplements.htm. Or you can create your own using the herbs mentioned in chapter 8. Another option is to buy a preformulated cleansing formula from a reliable source like Herb-Pharm or Gaia.

3. Introduce one of the breathing exercises in appendix B into your life. Perform it daily.

4. Start the diet plan described in chapter 9.

5. Perform the meridian stretches described in appendix A. These stretches restore balance and circulation in the body. You can do

them first thing in the morning when you wake up or before you go to bed. Choose the time that works best for you. They won't take more than five minutes of your time.

WEEK 2

On week two, you will continue the same actions as week one. The idea is to give you time to adjust to all the changes you are making.

1. Continue with symptom management and again try to see if you can replace medicine with an herbal supplement.
2. Continue taking detox herbal supplements.
3. Continue doing one of the breathing exercises in appendix B daily.
4. Continue with the diet plan described in chapter 9.
5. Continue doing the meridian stretches described in appendix A.

WEEK 3

On week three, you will continue to cleanse and nourish. However, your body should be a little bit stronger and less toxic. Therefore, we now can also start working on restoring your gut.

1. Continue with symptom management for the symptoms that have not subsided and again try to see if you can replace medicine with an herbal supplement.
2. Continue taking detox herbal supplement.
3. Add a digestive tea and antimicrobial tincture to your regimen. As with the detox herbal supplement, you can use the formulas that I have designed specifically for this program. You can find it on my website at https://www.moongazingapothecary.com/autoimmune-herbal-supplements.htm. Another option is for you to create your own using the herbs mentioned in chapter 10 or

buying a preformulated cleansing formula from a reliable source like Herb-Pharm or Gaia Herbs.

4. Add a probiotic formula to your daily regimen.
5. Continue doing one of the breathing exercises in appendix B daily.
6. Continue with the diet plan described in chapter 9.
7. Continue doing the meridian stretches described in appendix A.

WEEK 4

On week four, you will continue the same actions as week three. The idea this week is to give you time to adjust to all the changes you have been making the last three weeks. You should start feeling better by now. However, it is time to begin eliminating toxins in your home so you do not revert any progress you had made.

1. Continue with symptom management for the symptoms that have not subsided and again try to see if you can replace medicine with an herbal supplement.
2. Continue taking detox herbal supplement. (This will be your last week.)
3. Continue digestive tea and antimicrobial tincture.
4. Continue taking the probiotic formula to your daily regimen.
5. Continue doing one of the breathing exercises in appendix B daily.
6. Continue with the diet plan described in chapter 9.
7. Continue doing the meridian stretches described in appendix A.
8. If you do not have an exercise regimen in place, introduce a thirty-minute walk every day of the week.
9. Make a list of all the toxic items in your household you need to eliminate (shampoos, cosmetics, and so on). Select one or two things and replace them with a cleaner alternative. *Optional*: If you

are up for it, eliminate more than two things from your household. Replace as many as you can without becoming overwhelmed emotionally or financially.

WEEK 5

Unless you have been sick for many years, have a severe health condition, or haven't been following the diet on chapter 9, by week five, you won't need the cleansing herbs anymore, and cleansing foods should be enough to continue to improve. You also should be feeling better physically. Therefore, we can focus on supporting your emotions. So you will be adding mindfulness meditation to your daily routine.

1. Continue with symptom management for the symptoms that have not subsided and again try to see if you can replace medicine with an herbal supplement. Depending on the medication, it is recommended to wean off conventional medicine before replacing it with a natural alternative, such as in the case as blood pressure and antidepressant meds.
2. Stop taking detox herbal supplement.
3. Continue digestive tea and antimicrobial tincture.
4. Continue taking the probiotic formula to your daily regimen.
5. Continue doing one of the breathing exercises in appendix B daily.
6. Continue with the diet plan described in chapter 9.
7. Continue doing the meridian stretches described in appendix A.
8. Continue exercising or take a thirty-minute walk every day of the week.
9. Select two or three more items from your list of toxic things in your household, and replace them with a cleaner alternative. *Optional*: Just like in week four, replace as many additional items as you can without becoming overwhelmed emotionally or financially.

10. Introduce mindfulness mediation described in appendix C. Choose a morning or evening to do it. It will only take a minute of your time. I recommend you do it right after stretching. This will create a routine.

WEEK 6

This week, you will continue with the program as previous weeks, and you will start assessing your nine environments (described in chapter 5) so you can begin making necessary changes to improve your quality of life. Do not get overwhelmed. You won't need to change all environments at once, and you will notice, as you change one environment, it will impact another for the better.

1. Unless you have a severe condition, are not following this program correctly, or have been ill for an extended period of time, you should see improvement, if not complete elimination of, your symptoms by now. If you still have symptoms, try to replace your medication with herbal supplements (unless your doctor advises you otherwise).
2. Continue digestive tea and antimicrobial tincture.
3. Continue taking the probiotic formula to your daily regimen.
4. Continue doing one of the breathing exercises in appendix B daily.
5. Continue with the diet plan described in chapter 9.
6. Continue doing the meridian stretches described in appendix A.
7. Continue exercising or take a thirty-minute walk every day of the week.
8. Select two or three more items from your list of toxic items in your household. Replace them with a cleaner alternative.
9. Continue mindfulness mediation described in appendix C.

10. One day this week, review the nine environments listed in chapter 5 and ask yourself, "What could I add, delete, or modify in each of these environments that would enhance the quality of my life?" or "What is irritating me?" Add whatever comes up to your list of toxic items to change. They can be small or large changes. For example, one of the first things I changed was from my physical environment. I got my garage door replaced. For five years, it only opened about ten inches when the temperature dropped below 62 degrees. (Fortunately that does not happen in California that often.) Every time it happened, I got angry and frustrated. What of a waste of energy on my part. Not only that, this affected my mood for part of my day. Such an easy solution! Fixing this item no longer affected my mood.

WEEK 7

By now, you should be way on your way with new healthy habits in place, such as meditation, stretching, proper diet, exercise, and so on. Now is time to add an adaptogen to help support your nervous system and adrenal glands.

1. Continue digestive tea and antimicrobial tincture.
2. Continue taking the probiotic formula to your daily regimen.
3. Add an adaptogen formula to your daily supplement intake. As with the detox herbal supplement, you can use the formula that I have designed specifically for this program. You can find it on my website at https://www.moongazingapothecary.com/autoimmune-herbal-supplements.htm. Or you can create your own using the herbs mentioned in chapter 10 or buy a preformulated adaptogen formula from a reliable source like Herb-Pharm or Gaia Herbs.
4. Continue doing one of the breathing exercises in appendix B daily.
5. Continue with the diet plan described in chapter 9.
6. Continue doing the meridian stretches described in appendix A.

7. Continue exercising or take a thirty-minute walk every day of the week.
8. Select two or three more items from your list of toxic items in your household. Replace them with a cleaner alternative.
9. Continue mindfulness mediation described in appendix C.

WEEK 8

On week eight, you will continue with your routine, including taking steps on improving one of your environments. You will also add a daily gratitude exercise to your daily routine. As you can see by now, these habits do not take too much of your time. Meditation, breathing exercises, stretching, and gratitude altogether take less than fifteen minutes, and the benefits outweigh the time you invest on them.

1. Continue digestive tea and antimicrobial tincture.
2. Continue taking the probiotic formula to your daily regimen.
3. Continue taking an adaptogen formula to your daily supplement intake.
4. Continue doing one of the breathing exercises in appendix B daily.
5. Continue with the diet plan described in chapter 9.
6. Continue doing the meridian stretches described in appendix A.
7. Continue exercising or take a thirty-minute walk every day of the week.
8. Select three or four more items from your list of toxic items or environmental changes that you need to do, and replace them with a better alternative.
9. Continue mindfulness mediation described in appendix C.

10. Start a gratitude journal by writing down each morning three things you are grateful for and three things you are looking forward to.

WEEK 9

No changes this week. Continue working as you did in week eight. You are almost at the end of the program. You are doing awesome, keep going!

1. Continue digestive tea and antimicrobial tincture.
2. Continue taking the probiotic formula to your daily regimen.
3. Continue taking an adaptogen formula to your daily supplement intake.
4. Continue doing one of the breathing exercises in appendix B daily.
5. Continue with the diet plan described in chapter 9.
6. Continue doing the meridian stretches described in appendix A.
7. Continue exercising or take a thirty-minute walk every day of the week.
8. Select three or four more items from your list of toxic items or environmental changes that you need to do, and replace them with a better alternative.
9. Continue mindfulness mediation described in appendix C.
10. Continue your gratitude journal. *Optional*: If you want to stretch yourself a little bit more, you can read and do the exercise in the book, *The Magic*, by Rhonda Byrne

WEEK 10

For week ten, you will continue working as you did in week nine. However, now you should feel better emotionally and be open to keep growing. Therefore, as an option, you can start working on finding a technique, book, or counselor to help you overcome limiting beliefs and increase your sense of self-love.

1. Continue digestive tea and antimicrobial tincture.
2. Continue taking the probiotic formula to your daily regimen.
3. Continue taking an adaptogen formula to your daily supplement intake.
4. Continue doing one of the breathing exercises in appendix B daily.
5. Continue with the diet plan described in chapter 9.
6. Continue doing the meridian stretches described in appendix A.
7. Continue exercising or take a thirty-minute walk every day of the week.
8. Select three or four more items from your list of toxic items or environmental changes that you need to do, and replace them with a better alternative.
9. Continue mindfulness mediation described in appendix C.
10. Continue your gratitude journal.
11. *Optional*: Find a book or a counselor that can help you replace limiting beliefs or improve your level of self-love. You can also use flower essences to help you with this.

WEEK 11

Congratulations on making this far! No changes this week. Continue working as you did in week ten.

1. Continue digestive tea and antimicrobial tincture.
2. Continue taking the probiotic formula to your daily regimen.
3. Continue taking an adaptogen formula to your daily supplement intake.

4. Continue doing one of the breathing exercises in appendix B daily.
5. Continue with the diet plan described in chapter 9.
6. Continue doing the meridian stretches described in appendix A.
7. Continue exercising or take a thirty-minute walk every day of the week.
8. Select three or four more items from your list of toxic items or environmental changes that you need to do, and replace them with a better alternative.
9. Continue mindfulness mediation described in appendix C.
10. Continue your gratitude journal.
11. *Optional*: Continue working on eliminating limiting beliefs or improving your level of self-love.

WEEK 12

You made it to the end of the basic program. Yay! No changes this week. Continue working as you did on week eleven.

1. Continue digestive tea and antimicrobial tincture.
2. Continue taking the probiotic formula to your daily regimen.
3. Continue taking an adaptogen formula to your daily supplement intake.
4. Continue doing one of the breathing exercises in appendix B daily.
5. Continue with the diet plan described in chapter 9.
6. Continue doing the meridian stretches described in appendix A.
7. Continue exercising or take a thirty-minute walk every day of the week.

8. Select three or four more items from your list of toxic items or environmental changes that you need to do, and replace them with a better alternative.
9. Continue mindfulness mediation described in appendix C.
10. Continue your gratitude journal.
11. *Optional*: Continue working on eliminating limiting beliefs or improve your level of self-love.

WEEK 13 (OPTIONAL)

If your symptoms have subsided, you can try start slowly reintroducing foods to your diet, such as gluten. However, you do not have to and are welcome to continue with the diet described in chapter 9. When reintroducing food, there are some exceptions:

- I do not recommend you ever add dairy back to your diet.
- Introduce only organic gluten and preferably only in non-processed form, such as wheat berries.
- Always avoid high amounts of caffeine, sugar, alcohol, and table salt (refined salt).
- Do your best to avoid toxic foods such as artificial sweeteners, coloring, GMO, high fructose corn syrup, trans fats, and hydrogenated fats.
- Always avoid food that you are allergic to.

Note that there is no right time to reintroduce foods, it varies from person to person. **Patience and method are the keys to a successful reintroduction**. Don't rush things by reintroducing several foods at the same time. If you do, you won't be able to distinguish which food may still be causing you problems. **It is crucial to reintroduce foods one at a time, following a** specific step-by-step process:

- Reintroduce one food at a time.

- Consume the food several times a day for three or four days
- Stop and continue the diet in chapter 9 for at least three days before reintroducing another food.
- If you have a reaction to the food you introduced, *stop eating that food*. Wait until symptoms subside before you reintroduce a new food. The following are symptoms you should look out for when reintroducing a food: Brain fog, depression/anxiety, digestive issues such as diarrhea, constipation gas or bloating, problems sleeping, fatigue, headache, emotional sensitivity or mood swings, joint pain, rashes, sleepiness or feeling tire after eating.

This week you can also stop or minimize the cleansing foods such as the cilantro juice and start moving toward the maintenance diet described on the last page of chapter 9. *Only do this if you are symptom-free*. For most people, this is an excellent time to start. However, even if you are better or if you still have symptoms with week thirteen, do the same as week twelve until you feel better.

1. Continue digestive tea and antimicrobial tincture.
2. Continue taking the probiotic formula to your daily regimen.
3. Continue taking an adaptogen formula to your daily supplement intake.
4. Continue doing one of the breathing exercises in appendix B daily.
5. Continue with the diet plan described in chapter 9.
6. Continue doing the meridian stretches described in appendix A.
7. Continue exercising or 30-minute walk every day of the week.
8. Select three or four more items from your list of toxic items or environmental changes that you need to do, and replace them with a better alternative.
9. Continue mindfulness mediation described in appendix C.
10. Continue your gratitude journal.

11. *Optional*: continue working on eliminating limiting beliefs or improving your level of self-love.

If you are wondering how long you should continue following this program, the answer is until you are healthy again. Please note that it took years to get to where you are; therefore, even if you feel better, it might take years to recover fully. I have seen with my clients that treatment usually takes between three and six months, assuming they follow this program every day. However, people with serious conditions may take between eighteen and twenty-four months to fully recover.

Regardless of your current health status, following the recommendations of this book will promote health and overall well-being. I recommend keeping as a daily routine all the stress management techniques, including meditation, the breathing exercises, and meridian stretches. Once you recovered or if you are currently healthy, you can cleanse twice a year using the diet in chapter 9 for two weeks and taking the herbal detox supplement as a prevention measure against illnesses.

It is crucial that you understand that your diagnosis does not define you, has not broken you, and cannot control you. The power to heal is within you. Lasting change does not just happen, it happens when you change your life, and this takes time, but it does not take a lot of effort or a long period of time to see vast improvements. Therefore, always remember the words of Robert Holden, "You are not your struggles. You are not your diagnosis. You are not your traumatic experiences. You are not broken." Remember to be kind, loving and patient with yourself throughout this process. Loving yourself is paramount, and the more you can tap into this the more vibrant your state of wellness will be.

Finally, take it a day at a time, be responsible for your life and take action. The sooner you can start living in the now and acting, the sooner you can start the recovery process.

APPENDIX A

Five Element Meridian Stretches

Meridian stretching is a method developed by Shiatsu therapist, Shizuto Masunaga. It is a yoga-like system, with a vast array of movements and stretches to be practiced with the intention of using them to restore balance and circulation in the body.

These stretches tonify each meridian pair and improve organ function, energy flow, and emotions. The goal is to relieve tightness, not to force yourself beyond what is comfortable and then feel pain. The more you practice, the more comfortable they become and the higher the effect on well-being and disease prevention.

1. Water Element

Kidney and Bladder Meridians

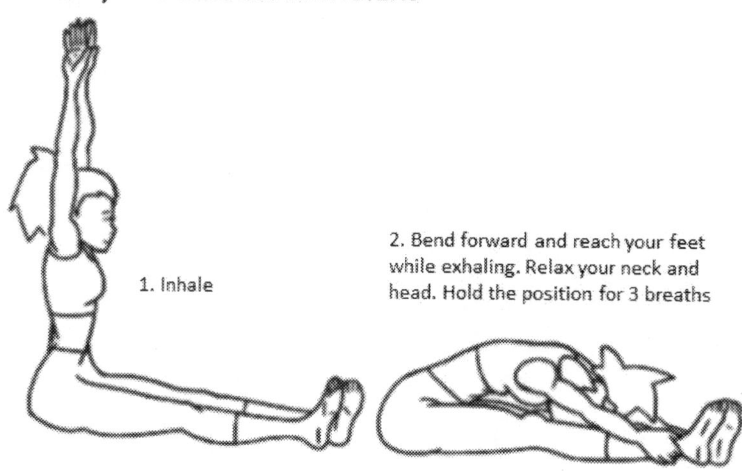

2. Wood Element Stretches

Liver and Gall bladder meridians

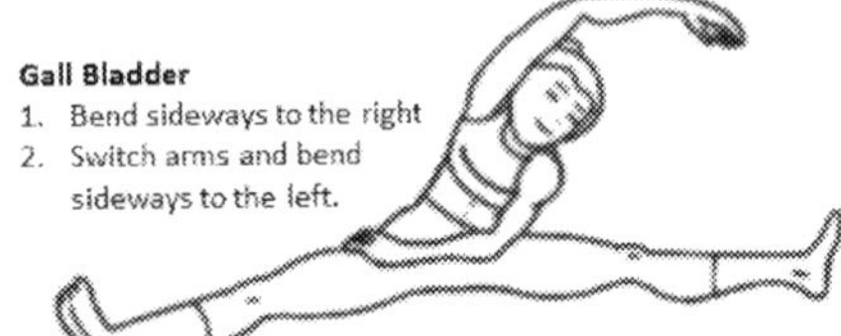

Gall Bladder

1. Bend sideways to the right
2. Switch arms and bend sideways to the left.

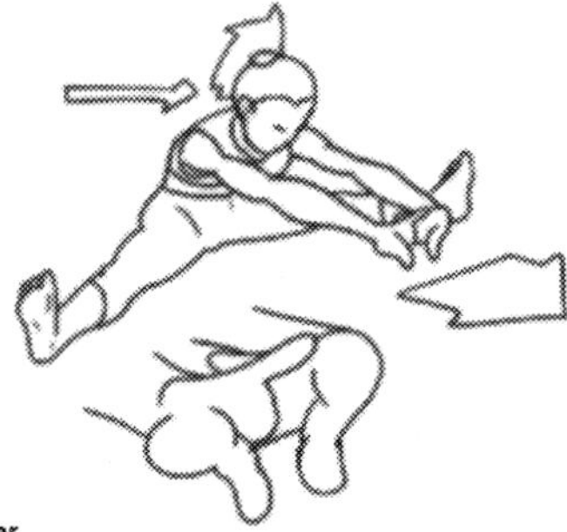

Liver

1. Interlace fingers of both hands together and turn hands so palms face outwards.
2. Bend forward from the hips as you extend arms forward

3. Fire Element Stretches

Pericardium and triple heater meridians

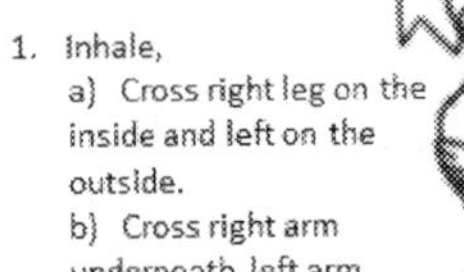

1. Inhale,
   a) Cross right leg on the inside and left on the outside.
   b) Cross right arm underneath left arm

2. Exhale while bending forward from the hips. When you reach a comfortable stretch, hold the position for 3 breaths.

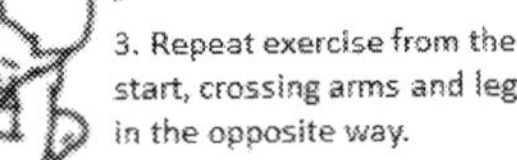

3. Repeat exercise from the start, crossing arms and legs in the opposite way.

Stomach and Small Intestine Meridians

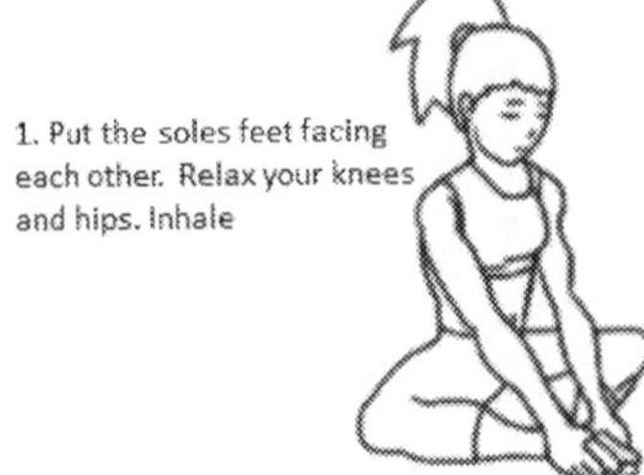

1. Put the soles feet facing each other. Relax your knees and hips. Inhale

2. Bend forward on exhaling. When you reach a comfortable stretch, hold the positions for 3 breaths.

4. Earth Element Stretches

Stomach and Spleen Meridians

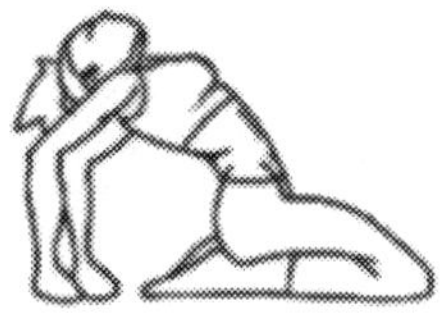

1. Inhale, relaxing your head back.

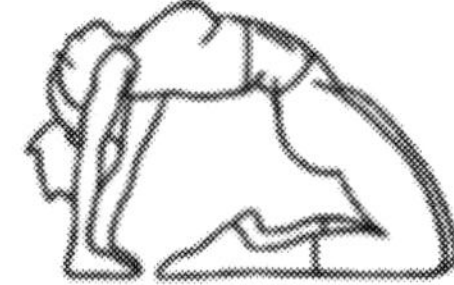

2. Exhale as you lift your hips up. Hold this position for 3 breaths into the abdomen.

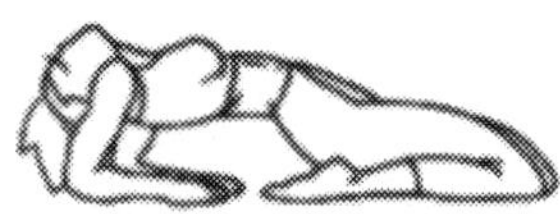

3. You can stretch more by leaning on your elbows for another 3 breaths.

5. Metal Element Stretches

Lungs and Large intestine meridians

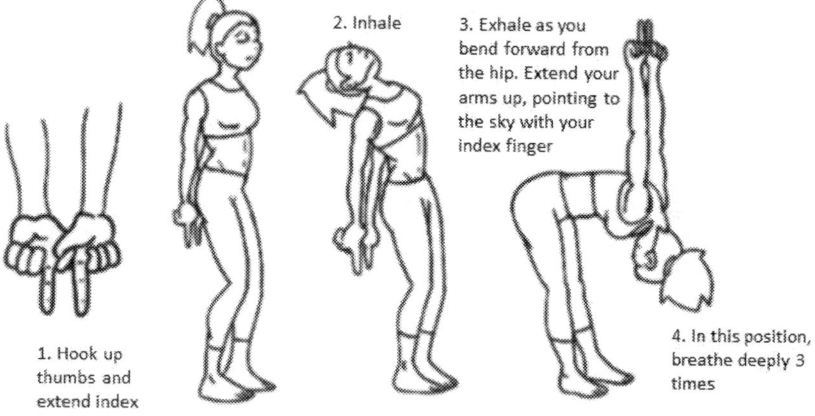

1. Hook up thumbs and extend index fingers

2. Inhale

3. Exhale as you bend forward from the hip. Extend your arms up, pointing to the sky with your index finger

4. In this position, breathe deeply 3 times

APPENDIX B
Deep Breathing Exercises

BREATHING EXERCISE #1

This is a straightforward exercise that can be done while sitting on the sofa, watching TV, or having a conversation with family or a friend. All you have to do is hold your hands behind your neck or behind your head, and hold that position for two or five minutes.

Sounds weird? Well, this exercise is based on science. Researchers found that, when people hold their arms at shoulder height, oxygen consumption and air intake are higher compared to when individuals hold their arms at their sides. The study showed that the benefits lasted for two minutes after the arms were lowered.

BREATHING EXERCISE #2

First thing in the morning when you wake up and at the end of the day before going to bed, place the tip of your tongue against the ridge behind your upper teeth and exhale completely through your mouth so you make a whoosh sound. Close your mouth and inhale deeply through your nose for a count of four, hold your breath for seven counts, and then exhale through your mouth for a count of eight. Repeat three times.

APPENDIX C

Mindfulness Meditation

MINDFUL BREATHING

This meditation can be done standing up or sitting down, at any time and any place. All you have to do is be still and focus on your breath for just one minute.

Start by breathing in and out slowly. One breath cycle should last for approximately four to six seconds. Breathe in through your nose and out through your mouth, letting your breath flow effortlessly in and out of your body. Purposefully watch your breath, focusing your sense of awareness on its pathway as it enters your body and exits the body and dissipates into the world.

Let go of any thoughts that come. Let go of things you have to do later today or pending work that need your attention. Simply focus on your breath, when you notice that you are thinking and no longer focused on your breath. Say the word *thinking*. Let go of the thought without any judgement or condemnation of the experience. Stay with whatever feeling arises, and go back to focusing on the breath.

In the advanced version of this exercise, when you notice that you are thinking, let go of the thought and connect with the emotion, the feeling. Process the emotion and ask yourself, "Who am I without these thoughts?"

It is important to note that mindfulness meditation is not about escaping, ignoring, or repressing negative emotions. Many people, including long-time practitioners of mediation, use meditation as a form of escaping difficult emotions. Meditation is about being present and experiencing whatever emotion arises without judgement and without chasing thoughts (rumination). It is about building awareness, feeling, and letting go of the judgment.

APPENDIX D
The Total Truth Letter

This is a technique I learned from Jack Canfield, and I have been using successfully for years. You can use the total truth letter to help you get you through difficult feelings or emotions. It is useful to release old resentments or if you have residual pain or incompleteness with a relationship in the present or the past.

Jack says the reason why this process works is because

> often, when we're upset, we fail to communicate all our true feelings to the person we're in conflict with. We get stuck at the point of anger or pain, and rarely move past it to emotional "completion." As a result, it can be difficult to feel close to—or even at ease with—the other person following such an angry or painful confrontation.

This process will help you express your true feelings without confrontation and at the end to take responsibility of your feelings once they are fully experienced and expressed.

PROCESS

Write a letter to the person who has upset you, with roughly equal portions of the letter expressing each of the following feelings

1. Anger and resentment

   I'm angry that … I'm fed up with …

   I hate it when … I resent …

I don't like it when … I can't stand …

2. Hurt

   It hurt me when … I feel awful about …

   I feel hurt that … I was heartbroken when …

   I feel sad when … I feel disappointed about …

3. Fear

   I was afraid that … I get afraid of you when …

   I feel scared when … I'm afraid that I …

4. Remorse, regret, accountability

   I'm sorry that … I'm sorry for …

   Please forgive me for … I didn't mean to …

5. Wants

   All I ever want(ed) … I want(ed) …

   I want you to … I deserve …

6. Love, Compassion, Forgiveness, Appreciation

   I understand that … Thank you for …

   I appreciate … I love you when …

   I love you because … I forgive you for …

   And I forgive myself for …

Destroy the letter once you have completed it. Remember, the main purpose is to get you free from the unexpressed emotions not to dump all your negative emotions on another person.

To learn more about Jack Canfield's work, visit www.JackCanfield.com

APPENDIX E

The Feeling Exercise

(Adapted from the feeling exercise from Arnold Patent)

As discussed in chapter 13, emotions are feelings distorted by thoughts, beliefs and expectations attached to those feelings. The process of reconnecting to our feelings requires a high level of intention and willingness to first feel our feelings just as they are without the fears and beliefs that suppressed them to begin with. The feeling exercise supports this process. Whenever you notice that a situation or feeling is bringing discomfort:

- Close your eyes and scan your body. Notice how you are feeling.
- Feel the feeling free of any thoughts or judgments. Feel the energy, the power, in the feeling.
- Let go of any thoughts that come up without judging them.
- As you begin the process of feeling your feelings without labels, descriptions or judgments, notice the energy in the feeling; The vibration in the feeling, the intensity of the vibration as it flows thru your body. Feel the intensity of this energy as power; your own power.
- Feel the love for the feeling just the way it is. Feel love for the power in the feeling.
- Feel love for yourself feeling the feeling and feeling the power of the feeling.

The second part of this exercise is an option, and it is useful when the emotions that you are feeling are triggered by a person. First, let yourself feel whatever feelings you have without judgment and follow the exercise above. When you get to a point where you can feel love for these feelings and yourself feeling them, bring your attention to anyone or anything that is causing the discomfort – be it your friend, partner, job, or employee, then:

- Ask your inner Self to assist you in feeling the feelings that are connected to these judgments. Feel the feelings as deeply as you can.
- Ask your inner Self to assist you in feeling the love for these feelings. Allow your heart to open and embrace these feelings.
- Feel deep love for your inner Self.
- Ask your inner Self to assist you in feeling forgiveness for this person. Allow your heart to open as wide as you can.
- Let this feeling of forgiveness expand into a deep love for this person. When you are ready, embrace the person in this deeply felt, open-hearted love.
- Feel the connection between you.

As you move to a place of feeling love for the person or situation, you will not only be relating to them heart to heart but you will feel more peaceful, and you will easily release the illusion of this being a problem.

ENDNOTES

1 Iris F. F. Benzie and Sissi Wachtel-Galor, *Herbal Medicine: Biomolecular and Clinical Aspects*, 2nd ed. (CRC Press/Taylor & Francis, 2011).
2 Candice Pert, PhD, *Molecules of Emotions* (New York: Touchstone, 1997).
3 Blair Justice, PhD, *Who gets Sick?* (Texas: PeAK Press, 2000).
4 Mario F. Fraga et al., "Epigenetic differences arise during the lifetime of monozygotic twins," *Proceedings of the National Academy of Sciences of the United States of America* 102 (30)(2005), 10604–10609.
5 Gary Marcus, PhD, "Making the Mind," *Boston Review* (December 2013).
6 Seymour Koblin, *Food for Life: Applying Macrobiotic Principles and Practice to Create Vital Health for Body, Mind and Spirit* (San Diego: Soul Star Creations, 1998).
7 Clemens Arvay, *The Biophilia Effect: A Scientific and Spiritual Exploration of the Healing Bond Between Humans and Nature* (Sounds True, 2018).
8 Martin A. Makary, "Medical error-the third leading cause of death in the US," *BMJ*, May 3, 2016.
9 Gary Null, PhD, et al., "Death by Medicine," *Journal of Orthomolecular Medicine* 20 (2005).
10 Michael Barry, *The Forgiveness Project: The Startling Discovery of How to Overcome Cancer, Find Health, and Achieve Peace* (Grand Rapids: Kregel Publications, 2011).
11 Paul Gilbert, *The Compassionate Mind* (New Harbinger Publications, Inc., 2009).
12 Kemerling, *Aristotle: Ethics and the Virtues* (2001).
13 Jonathan Haidt, *The Happiness Hypothesis* (New York: Basic Books, 2006).
14 Deborah D. Danner, David A. Snowdon, and Wallace V. Friesen, "Positive Emotions in Early Life and Longevity: Findings from the Nun Study," *Journal of Personality and Social Psychology* (2000).
15 Martin E. P. Seligman, *Authentic Happiness: Using the New Positive Psychology to Realize Your Potential for Lasting Fulfillment* (New York: Free Press, 2002).

16 S. Lyubomirsky, L. A. King, and E. Diener, "The benefits and costs of frequent positive affect: Does happiness lead to success?" *Psychological Bulletin* (2005).
17 Dian Land, "Study shows compassion meditation changes the brain" (2008).
18 R. Hernandez et al., "Optimism and Cardiovascular Health: Optimism and Cardiovascular Health: Multi-Ethnic Study of Atherosclerosis (MESA)," *Health Behavior and Policy Review* 2(1), 2015, 62–73.
19 Norman Shealy, MD, PhD. *Life Beyond 100* (London: Pinguin Group, 2005).
20 K. Pettingall, "Mental attitudes to cancer: an additional prognostic factor," *Lancet* (1990), 750.
21 S. Green, "Psychological response to breast cancer and 15 year outcome," *Lancet* (1990), 49–50.
22 Andrew Weil, "Attitude is everything with aging," *Andrew Weil Self Healing Newsletter* (September 2006).
23 N. Digdon and A. Koble, "Effects of Constructive Worry, Imagery Distraction, and Gratitude Interventions on Sleep Quality: A Pilot Trial," *Applied Psychology: Health and Wellbeing* (May 2011).
24 P. L. Hill, M. Allemand, and B. W. Roberts, "Examining the Pathways between Gratitude and Self-Rated Physical Health across Adulthood," *Journal of the International Society for the Study of Individual Differences* (January 2013), 92–96.
25 T. B. Kashdan, G. Uswatte, and T. Julian, "Gratitude and hedonic and eudaimonic well-being in Vietnam war veterans," *Behavior Research and Therapy* (February 2006), 177–199.
26 B. L. Fredrickson et al., "What good are positive emotions in crisis? A prospective study of resilience and emotions following the terrorist attacks on the United States on September 11th, 2001," *Journal of Personality and Social Psychology* (2003), 365–376.
27 L. Redwine, "A pilot randomized study of a gratitude journaling intervention on HRV and inflammatory biomarkers in Stage B heart failure patients," *Psychosomatic Medicine* (2016), 667–676.
28 S. T. Cheng, P. K. Tsui, and J. H. Lam, "Improving mental health in health care practitioners: randomized controlled trial of a gratitude intervention," *PsychInfo Database* (September 14, 2014), 177–186.
29 Robert A. Emmons, *The Little Book of Gratitude* (Great Britain: Gaia Books, 2016).
30 Giacomo Rizzolatti and Laila Craighero, "Mirror Neuron: a neurological approach to empathy," *Journal of Neurobiology of Human Values* (2005).
31 Marc Barasch, *The Compassionate Life: Walking the Path of Kindness* (Berret-Koehler Publishers, Inc., 2009).

32 E. Diener, "Happy People Live Longer: Subjective well-being contributes to health and longevity," *Applied Psychology: Health and Well-being* (2011).
33 HH The Dalai Lama and Dr. Howard Cutler, *The Art of Happiness* (New York: Riverhead Books, 1998).
34 HH The Dalai Lama, *The Compassionate Life* (Massachusetts: Wisdom Publications, Inc., 2003).
35 Hart, *Living Oneness. Global Oneness Project* (2005).
36 Dacher Keltner, "Darwin's Touch: Survival of the Kindest," http://www.psychologytoday.com/blog/born-be-good/200902/darwins-touch-survival-the-kindest.
37 Sonja Lyubomirsky, *The How of Happiness: A Scientific Approach to Getting the Life You Want* (New York: Penguin Press, 2008).
38 Paul J. Zak, Angela Stanton, and Sheila Ahmadi. "Oxytocin Increases Generosity in Humans," *PLoS ONE Journal* (2007).
39 R. Veenhoven, *Healthy Happiness, Journal of Happiness Studies* 9 (2008), 449–469.
40 Harvard, Kennedy School. *Social Capital Community Benchmark Survey* (2006).
41 Jorge Moll et al., "Human Fronto-mesolimbic networks guide descisions about charitable donation," (National Institute of Health, 2006).
42 R. J. Davidson and A. Lutz, "Buddha's Brain: Neuroplasticity and Meditation," *IEEE Signal Processing Magazine* (25)(1), 176–174.
43 Lorne Ladner, PhD, *The Lost Art of Compassion: Discovering the Practice of Happiness in the Meeting of Buddhism and Psychology* (New York: HarperCollins, 2004).
44 Pew Research Center Religion & Public Life, "Highly religious Americans are happier and more involved with family but are no more likely to exercise, recycle or make socially conscious consumer choices," (April 2016).
45 Harvard, Women's Health Watch, "Attending religious services linked to longer lives, study shows," (Harvard Health Publishing, 2016).
46 Lisa Miller et al., "Neuroanatomical Correlates of Religiosity and Spirituality," *JAMA Psychiatry* (2013).
47 Harold G. Koenig, "Association of Religious Involvement and Suicide," *JAMA Psychiatry* (2016).
48 American Psychological Association, "Religion or spirituality has positive impact on romantic/marital relationships, child development, research shows," ScienceDaily (2014).
49 Pew Research Center, "Highly religious Americans are more satisfied with their family life," *Religion & Public Life* (2016).
50 Codie R Rouleau, Sheila N. Garland, and Linda E. Carlson, "The impact of mindfulness-based interventions on symptom burden, positive psychological

outcomes, and biomarkers in cancer patients," *Cancer Management and Research* (7)(2015), 121–131.

51 M. W. Taal and B. M. Brenner, "Evolving strategies for renoprotection: non-diabetic chronic renal disease," *Current Opinion in Nephrology and Hypertension* 10(4)(July 2001), 523–531.

52 R. Swaminathan, "Nutritional factors in osteoporosis," *International Journal of Clinical Practices* 53(7)(October-November 1999), 540–548.

53 A. Samsel and S. Seneff, "Glyphosate, pathways to modern diseases II: Celiac sprue and gluten intolerance," *Interdisciplinary Toxicology* 6(4)(2013), 159–184.

54 Paul Pitchford, *Healing with Whole Foods* (Berkeley, Calif.: North Atlantic Books, 2002).

55 C. Snell et al., "Assessment of the health impact of GM plant diets in long-term and multigenerational animal feeding trials: a literature review," *Food and Chemical Toxicology* 50(3–4)(March 2012), 1134–1148.

56 Herman Aihara, *Acid and Alkaline*, 5th ed. (George Ohsawa Macrobiotic, 1986).

57 Steve Gagne, *The Energetics of Foods* (Rochester: Healing Arts Press, 1990).

58 Benjamin P. Chapman, "Emotion suppression and mortality risk over a 12-year follow-up," *Journal of Psychosomatic Research* 75, 381–385.

59 Centers for Disease Control and Prevention, "Chronic Diease Prevention and Health Promotion," https://www.cdc.gov/chronicdisease/overview/index.htm.

60 U.S. Department of Health and Human Services Office on Women's Health, *Autoimmune Diseases Fact Sheet* (2012).

61 WorldOmeters, "The United States Population (Live)," Department of Economic and Social Affairs, Population Division, May 30, 2018.

62 S. M. Rappaport, "Discovering environmental causes of disease," *Journal of Epidemiol Community Health* 66(2), 99–102.

63 A. Vojdani, K. M. Pollard, and A. W. Campbell, "Environmental Triggers and Autoimmunity," National Institute of Health 798029.

64 V. Molina and Y. Shoenfeld, "Infection, vaccines and other environmental triggers of autoimmunity," *National Institute of Health—Autoimmunity* 38(3), 235–245.

65 J. F. de Carvalho, R. M. Pereira, and Y. Shoenfeld, "The mosaic of autoimmunity: the role of environmental factors," *Front Biosci* (June 1, 2009), 501–509.

66 Andrew W. Campbell, "Autoimmunity and the Gut," Hindawi Publishing Corporation—Autoimmune Diseases, 12.

67 Pesticide Action Network, "Monsanto and Co.'s Dirty Little Secret."

68 Benoit Chassaing et al., "Dietary emulsifiers impact the mouse gut microbiota promoting colitis and metabolic syndrome," *International Journal of Science* 519 (2015), 92–96.

69 "Consumption of ultra-processed foods and cancer risk: results from NutriNet-Santé prospective cohort," *BMJ* 360 (2018), 322.

70 I. Delimaris, "Adverse Effects Associated with Protein Intake above the Recommended Dietary Allowance for Adults," *ISRN Nutrition* 126929 (2013).

71 Rahul Ray et al., "Effect of Dietary Vitamin D and Calcium on the Growth of Androgen-insensitive Human Prostate Tumor in a Murine Model," Anticancer Research 32(3)(2012), 727–731.

72 National Institute of Cancer at the National Institutes of Health, "Calcium and Cancer Prevention," https://www.cancer.gov/about-cancer/causes-prevention/risk/diet/calcium-fact-sheet.

73 J. Holt-Lunstad and T. B. Smith, "Loneliness and social isolation as risk factors for CVD: implications for evidence-based patient care and scientific inquiry," *Heart* 102(13)(July 2016), 987–989.

74 C. Wrosch, "Regret intensity, diurnal cortisol secretion, and physical health in older individuals: Evidence for directional effects and protective factors," *Psychology and Aging* 22(2007), 319–330.

75 Institute of HeartMath, "The Making of Emotions," https://www.heartmath.org/articles-of-the-heart/science-of-the-heart/making-emotions.

76 S. N. Yang, "The Effects of Environmental Toxins on Allergic Inflammation," *Allergy, Asthma & Immunology Research* 6(6)(2014), 478–484.

77 E. K. Leffel, "Drinking water exposure to cadmium, an environmental contaminant, results in the exacerbation of autoimmune disease in the murine model," *Toxicology* 188 (2003), 233–250.

78 Karen Feldscher, "High levels of fluorinated compounds have been linked to cancer, hormone disruption," *The Harvard Gazette* (2016).

79 N. Brautbar, A. Campbell, and A. Vojdani, "Silicone breast implants and autoimmunity: causation, association, or myth?" *J Biomater Sci Polym* 7(2) (1995), 133–145.

80 Graham C. L. Davey, PhD, "Negative news on TV is increasing, but what are its psychological effects?" *Psychology Today*, https://www.psychologytoday.com/us/blog/why-we-worry/201206/the-psychological-effects-tv-news.

81 World Health Organization (WHO), *Report of WHO global survey* (Geneva: National Policy on Traditional Medicine and Regulation of Herbal Medicine, 2005).

82 National Institute of Health, National Center for Complementary and Integrative Health, https://nccih.nih.gov/research/statistics/NHIS.

83 M. F. E. Chan et al., "Attitudes of Hong Kong Chinese to traditional Chinese medicine and Western medicine: Survey and cluster analysis," *Complement Ther Med* 11(2)(2003), 103–109.

84 Roger Ulrich, "View Through a Window May Influence Recovery from Surgery," *Science* 224, 420–421.

85 Yoshinori Ohtsuka, "Effects of forest environments on blood glucose," NOVA Biomedical (2003), 111–116.

86 Bum-Jin Park, "Effect of the forest environment on physiological relaxation using the results of field tests at 35 sites throughout Japan," *Forest Medicine* (2013), 57–67.

87 Jack Canfield, "Taking Control of the Environments that Control You," http://jackcanfield.com/blog/taking-control-of-the-environments-that-control-you.

88 The Foundation for Inner Peace, *Course in Miracles* (Mill Valley: 2007).

89 The Power of Positivity, "8 Studies that Show How Consciousness Affects Reality," https://www.powerofpositivity.com/8-studies-show-consciousness-affects-reality.

90 S. A. Hooker, K. S. Masters, and C. L. Park, "A meaningful life is a healthy life: a conceptual model linking meaning and meaning salience to health," *Review of General Psychology* (July 6, 2017).

91 James L. Wilson, *Adrenal Fatigue: The 21st Century Stress Syndrome* (Petaluma: Smart Publications, 2001).

92 David Winston and Steven Maimes, *Adaptogens: Herbs for Strength, Stamina, and Stress Relief* (Rochester: Healing Arts Press, 2007).

93 I. Solhaug et al., "Medical and Psychology Student's Experiences in Learning Mindfulness: Benefits, Paradoxes, and Pitfalls," *Mindfulness* (April 6, 2016), 838–850.

94 Diana Coholic, Mark Eys, and Sean Lougheed, "Investigating the Effectiveness of an Arts-Based and Mindfulness-Based Group Program for the Improvement of Resilience in Children in Need," *Journal of Child and Family Studies* 21(5)(October 2011).

95 J. Randye Semple et al., "A Randomized Trial of Mindfulness-Based Cognitive Therapy for Children: Promoting Mindful Attention to Enhance Social-Emotional Resiliency in Children," *Journal of Child and Family Studies* 19 (April 2010), 218–229.

96 Phillippa Lally et al., "How are habits formed: Modelling habit formation in the real world," *European Journal of Social Psychology* (2009).

97 Robert W. Firestone, PhD, "You Don't Really Know Yourself: Examining the persistence of our negative self-identity," https://www.psychologytoday.com/us/blog/the-human-experience/201611/you-dont-really-know-yourself.

98 Andy Martens, Jeff Greenberg, and John J. B. Allen, "Self-Esteem and Autonomic Physiology: Parallels Between Self-Esteem and Cardiac Vagal Tone as Buffers of Threat," *Journal of Research in Personality* 12, 370–389.

99 Kristin Neff, *Self-Compassion: The Proven Power of Being Kind to Yourself* (New York : HarperCollins, 2011).

100 Routledge, *From Aristotle to Augustine: Routledge History of Philosophy*, vol. 2 (London: 2003).

101 Amelia Karraker, Robert F.Schoeni, and Jennifer C. Cornman, "Psychological and cognitive determinants of mortality: Evidence from a nationally representative sample followed over thirty-five years," *Social Science & Medicine* 144 (November 2015), 69–78.

102 E. Mostofsky, E. A. Penner, M. A. Mittleman, "Outbursts of anger as a trigger of acute cardiovascular events: a systematic review and meta-analysis," *European Heart Journal* 1;35(21)(June 2014), 1404–1410.

103 P. M. Barnes, B. Bloom, and R. Nahin, "Complementary and alternative medicine use among adults and children," *CDC National Health Statistics Report* 12 (November 5, 2008).

104 Derek D. Rucker and Adam D. Galinsky, "Desire to Acquire: Powerlessness and compensatory consumption," https://insight.kellogg.northwestern.edu/article/desire_to_acquire.

105 Mary Beth Pinto, Phylis M. Mansfield, and Diane H. Parente, "Relationship of Credit Attitude and Debt to Self-Esteem and Locus of Control in College-Age Consumers," *Penn State Erie* 94 (June 1, 2004), 1405

INDEX

B

C

D

E

F

G

H

N

O

P

Q

R

S

T

U

V

W

Printed in the United States
by Baker & Taylor Publisher Services